Managing Clinical Problems in

Managing Clinical Problems in Diabetes

Edited by

Trisha Dunning
AM, RN, MEd, PhD, CDE, FRCNA

Glenn Ward
MBBS, BSc, DPhil (Oxon), FRACP, FRCPath

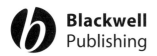

Blackwell Publishing editorial offices:
Blackwell Publishing Ltd, 9600 Garsington Road, Oxford OX4 2DQ, UK
  Tel: +44 (0)1865 776868
Blackwell Publishing Inc., 350 Main Street, Malden, MA 02148-5020, USA
  Tel: +1 781 388 8250
Blackwell Publishing Asia Pty Ltd, 550 Swanston Street, Carlton, Victoria 3053, Australia
  Tel: +61 (0)3 8359 1011

First published 2008 by Blackwell Publishing Ltd

ISBN: 9781405155717

Library of Congress Cataloging-in-Publication Data
Managing clinical problems in diabetes / edited by Trisha Dunning, Glenn Ward.
    p. ; cm.
  Includes bibliographical references and index.
  ISBN-13: 978-1-4051-5571-7 (pbk. : alk. paper)
  ISBN-10: 1-4051-5571-X (pbk. : alk. paper)
1. Diabetes–Treatment.   2. Diabetes–Complications–Treatment.   I. Dunning, Trisha.
II. Ward, Glenn, MBBS.
[DNLM: 1. Diabetes Mellitus–therapy–Case Reports. WK 815 M2654 2008]
RC660.M338 2008
616.4′6206–dc22

                                                                    2007029631

A catalogue record for this title is available from the British Library

Set in 11/13 Sabon by Graphicraft Limited, Hong Kong
Printed and bound in Singapore by C.O.S. Printers Pte Ltd

The publisher's policy is to use permanent paper from mills that operate a sustainable
forestry policy, and which has been manufactured from pulp processed using acid-free
and elementary chlorine-free practices. Furthermore, the publisher ensures that the text
paper and cover board used have met acceptable environmental accreditation standards.

For further information on Blackwell Publishing, visit our website:
www.blackwellnursing.com

Contents

Author profiles

Editors

Trisha Dunning
AM, RN, MEd, PhD, CDE, FRCNA

Professor Dunning is the Inaugural Chair in Nursing at Deakin University and Barwon Health in Victoria, Australia. She has been a diabetes educator for 20 years and is passionate about holistic nursing care. Trisha is the Inaugural Chair of the International Diabetes Federation (IDF) Consultative Section on Diabetes Education. She is the author of several books for people with diabetes and many books and papers for health professionals. She is an active researcher with a focus on people's beliefs and attitudes and how they affect professional care and self-care. Trisha is a very active worker on a great many Australian and international diabetes-related committees.

Glenn Ward
MBBS, BSc, DPhil (Oxon), FRACP, FRCPath

Glenn Ward is Head of Diabetes Services and Deputy Director, Department of Endocrinology and Diabetes, Clinical Consultant in the Department of Clinical Biochemistry at St. Vincent's Hospital, Melbourne, Australia. He is an Associate Professor in the University of Melbourne Department of Pathology, and a Senior Fellow, Clinical School University of Melbourne, St Vincent's Hospital. He was President of the Australian Diabetes Society from 2002–2004; Vice President of the Australian Diabetes Society 2000–2002; Chair of the Medical, Educational and Scientific Council of Diabetes Australia National 1998–2000; Honorary Secretary of the Australian Diabetes Society 1998–2000; a Councilor of the Australian Diabetes Society 1994–2004; Member of Board of Directors of Diabetes Australia

1994–2004; a Member of the National Executive Committee of Diabetes Australia 2002–2004; and is the current Chair of the Cross Cultural Committee of Diabetes Australia. Glenn has over 70 published articles focusing on in vivo research on insulin action and secretion in human subjects.

Contributors

Ralph Audehm
MBBS, DipRACOG, Graduate Certificate in Clinical Research

Ralph is a general practitioner in Melbourne with a special interest in diabetes education and care. He is the GP Liaison Officer with the Royal Melbourne Hospital and Medical Advisor to Diabetes Australia, Victoria. He is active on several local and state committees concerning diabetes and collaborates in research projects through the Department of General Practice, the University of Melbourne.

Thyra Bolton
EN

Thyra Bolton has coordinated the High-risk Foot Clinic at Royal Prince Alfred Hospital in Sydney since its inception in 1988. She has been extensively involved in health professional training, especially in rural areas and for visiting health professionals from overseas. Thyra has assisted in the establishment of high-risk foot clinics in Fiji and Thursday Island, which included training health professionals. Together with the staff of Royal Prince Alfred Diabetes Service she established the first High-risk Foot Telemedicine Service and continues to participate in online consultations. She was an invited speaker at the IDF Congress in Mexico in 2000 and Paris in 2003, the Vascular Conference in China in 2004 and contributed to the NSW *Better Practice Guidelines on the Management of Lower Limb Ulceration*.

Lesley Braun
B Pharm, Dip Appl Sci (Naturopathy), Grad Dip Phytotherapy

Lesley is a qualified pharmacist, naturopath, and herbalist. She acts as a consultant to industry and is a senior lecturer in The Australian College of Natural Medicine. Lesley is frequently invited to speak on complementary medicines. She is the author of many articles about natural medicines, and writes a regular column for the *Journal of Complementary Medicine*. She is the author of *Herbs and Natural Supplements*, which is now in its second edition.

Trudi Deakin
BSc (Hons), Ad Dip, PGCE, PhD, RD

Dr Trudi Deakin is Clinical Champion for the East Lancashire Diabetes Network and Chief Research Dietitian. Trudi qualified as a dietitian in 1993, specialised in paediatric diabetes in 1994 and became a diabetes specialist dietitian (adults/children) in 1996. Enrolment in a postgraduate certificate in education (PGCE) course enabled her to develop adult education principles. Concentrating on structured patient education, she undertook further research and was awarded a doctorate in diabetes in 2004. Trudi is passionate about researching, modernising and improving diabetes care and treatment and has assisted in developing and implementing many national initiatives. She is also an active member of the Diabetes UK Professional Advisory Council.

Sandra Hood
BSc (Hons), RD, DipADP

Sandra Hood is a specialist diabetes dietitian. She is the Lead for the Diabetes Service, working for the Nutrition and Dietetic Department, Dorset County Hospital, Dorchester, UK. She has a specialist interest in vegan diets and is an accomplished author and authority in this field. Since the recent changes in the management of diabetes care Sandra has developed a well-respected structured patient education programme.

Pamela Jones
RN, CDE

Pamela Jones is manager of the Diabetes Referral Centre at Barwon Health, the Geelong Hospital, Geelong, Victoria, Australia. Pamela is a Credentialed Diabetes Educator and has been working in diabetes since 1989. She has extensive experience working with children and adults with diabetes, both in the acute and community care setting.

Pamela was responsible for the establishment of the Barwon Region Diabetes Educator's working group in 1990. This group consists of multidisciplinary health professionals, who focus on sharing information and expertise that is aimed at improving client education. Pamela has a special interest in diabetes and pregnancy. This led to the development of a gestational diabetes ambulatory care programme that promotes women's potential for self-care with little disruption to their lives during this very special time. Pamela regularly conducts diabetes courses for nurses and other health professional and community groups.

Marg McGill
RN, MSc (Med)

Marg McGill has been a Vice President of the International Diabetes Federation (IDF) since 2003 and was appointed the Senior Vice President in 2006. Since 2000 she has been Chair of the IDF Consultative Section on Diabetes Education. In this role she has actively promoted the importance of role of the health professional. She has conducted leadership needs assessment workshops and professional education programmes in most regions of the IDF. She has led teams to develop (1) an International Curriculum for Diabetes Health Professional Education; (2) Content for the Curriculum; (3) an IDF-recognised Multidisciplinary Education Program for Diabetes Health Professionals; and (4) International Standards for Diabetes Education. She was Australia's first paediatric diabetes educator in 1978. For the last 18 years she has managed the Royal Prince Alfred Hospital Diabetes Ambulatory Care Centre, which is a large adult service focusing on clinical care and research. Her clinical and research interest is in the assessment and management of diabetic complications. She has published consistently on this topic in peer-reviewed journals. She is a regular invited speaker at many international diabetes scientific meetings.

Vanessa Nubé
Dip App Sci (Podiatry), MSc (Med)

Vanessa is senior podiatrist at the Royal Prince Alfred Hospital Diabetes Centre. In 2000 she was appointed co-ordinator of the Diabetes Amputation Prevention Programme for the Central Sydney Area Health Service, which introduces strategies for improving the management of diabetic foot disease. An invited speaker on the topic of diabetic foot disease both locally and internationally, Vanessa's publications include two original research papers published in *The Foot* and *The Journal of the American Podiatric Medical Association* and she has contributed to other publications on the diabetic foot including the NSW Health publication *Lower Limb Ulcers in People with Diabetes*. She is on the advisory committee for the *Australasian Journal of Podiatric Medicine*.

Michelle Robins
RN, MRCNA, Graduate Certificate in Diabetes Education, CDE

Michelle Robins is an endorsed nurse practitioner with 14 years' experience as a diabetes educator in a variety of settings. Her interests in diabetes management include improving the care of older people with diabetes, type 1 diabetes in young adults and better management strategies for people with type 2 diabetes who have complex needs. She is passionate about educating health professionals and building strong networks between the tertiary and primary care sectors.

Chas Skinner
Psychologist

Dr Chas Skinner was Senior Lecturer in Health Psychology, University of Southampton, UK, before taking up his current position at the University of Wollongong, NSW, Australia.

Victoria Stevenson
RN, FRCNA, CDE

Victoria is the Diabetes Clinical Nurse Coordinator at Austin Health, Victoria, Australia. In her many years in diabetes education, Victoria has established diabetes education services in several hospitals and a private diabetes education practice. She developed teaching resources that help people come to terms with the practicalities of having diabetes, and co produced several videos, the most recent being *Join with Us*, which promotes the Australian Diabetes Educators Association. Victoria is actively involved in state and national diabetes health professional groups that aim to better inform people with diabetes and those associated with them.

Sheridan Waldron
RD, BA, PhD

Sheridan is a specialist diabetes dietitian working for Dorset County Hospital, Dietetic Department. She has spent over 20 years working with children and adults with diabetes. Her research interests concern the dietary management of children's diabetes. Her current research is examining the barriers and facilitators of dietary change in children with type 1 diabetes. She has held national positions that have contributed to setting national recommendations and policy in the UK. She also holds official positions in the International Society for Pediatric and Adolescent Diabetes and the International Diabetes Federation.

Foreword

It is a great pleasure to pen the foreword to this significant book. Never was the presence of the contributing authors so strongly present, deeply courageous in the exposure of their personal and professional responses that in turn makes this book so highly engaging. It embodies a candour and integrity that goes beyond the contemporary constraining philosophy of political correctness and has at its heart the centrality of the patient and moves it into the principles and philosophy of what I call the humanity of care.

The structure, while logical, has the merit that the introduction of each of the eleven chapters is reflected in the reality of the referrals and the signature of key points. Each chapter is appropriately referenced and the principle of evidence base is critically followed and resonates in the response to the individual referrals. The authors have moved beyond the paradigm of acute management and are firmly embedded in the paradigm of chronic disease management.

Using the professional narrative approach from the perspective of different disciplines exemplifies the core constituents of a multidisciplinary professional team. While the approach may differ in some respects, the key elements of dialogue between the individual authors have resonance with the model of patient narrative as exemplified by Dr Natalia Piana *et al*. in the use of patient narrative in therapeutic patient education.

The examples and availability of actual referrals, professional or self referrals, give an authenticity and resonance for diabetes teams in daily practice. This is what makes this book so vibrant. It has the merit of promoting private reflection as well as team reflection. Furthermore, as an educational learning tool it has much to recommend by way of use for group discussion and it has additional merit in master class format for both specialists and non-specialists alike.

While the book can be read in one sitting it is also eminently suitable for use as a selective reference source for dipping into as needed and incorporated into structured professional education in the specialty of diabetes. It is of particular note that although the majority of the authors work in the Australian health care system there is a universality of message that diffuses into all health care systems.

The enduring imprint that this book leaves on me is the primacy of the patient and the imperative of multi-disciplinary and inter-disciplinary co-operation in managing clinical problems in diabetes and enabling individual patients to continue their journey of life-long self management.

Anne-Marie Felton
President, Federation of
European Nurses in Diabetes

Preface

The idea for this book grew out of a constant flow of telephone and email requests for advice, particularly from rural health professionals, and responding to letters from people with diabetes in a regular column in *Diabetes Conquest,* a magazine for people with diabetes. Many of our colleagues will recognise their patients in the case histories presented in the book. Obviously names have been withheld, identifying information removed, and the initials changed to protect the privacy of both the people with diabetes and their health professional carers.

Rationale for the book

The incidence and prevalence of diabetes is increasing globally. Therefore, most health professionals are likely to care for people with diabetes and often find they have to make clinical decisions without expert support, which can be difficult.

The proposed book aims to support theory with practical suggestions for addressing common clinical problems based on evidence and the clinical experience of diabetes educators, endocrinologists, general practitioners, and other health professionals who encounter such problems on a daily basis. The book was designed to be used as a clinical resource and illustrate how the health professionals concerned approach common clinical problems. It was also designed to complement other diabetes texts.

Aims of the book

The aims are to:

(1) address commonly encountered diabetes management problems;
(2) develop comprehensive responses from a range of relevant health professionals who suggest management approaches relevant to their area of practice. The specific health professionals who

provide comments about each case depend on the specific clinical issue; and

(3) stimulate thought and discussion.

Target readership

The target readership is health professionals from a range of professional backgrounds and general as well as specialist professionals such as general practitioners, nurses, dietitians, and podiatrists. The book will be particularly useful for beginner practitioners specialising in diabetes. In addition, it will provide suggestions or food for thought for more experienced practitioners.

The cases discussed in the book are all real and are presented exactly as the information was received from the person making the referral. General practitioners, diabetes educators and people with diabetes referred most of the cases; some were self-referrals by people with diabetes. They represent referrals to various diabetic health professionals and concern commonly encountered clinical issues. A list of key chapter points and recommended reading accompanies each chapter.

Trisha Dunning and Glenn Ward

Dedication and acknowledgements

This book is dedicated to all people with diabetes and the health professionals who care for them.

Glenn and I sincerely acknowledge the contributions of all the authors whose voices can be heard in this book for facing the challenge of suggesting management options for the cases presented and making their critical thinking, reflective practice, and problem-solving processes visible through those suggestions.

Diabetes management – a matter of balance

The essence of diabetes care is achieving balance in all aspects of the life of a person with diabetes. Achieving balance requires lifelong collaborative, multidisciplinary care where the person with diabetes plays a central role in determining his or her life priorities, health goals and planning his/her care. There is a 'doctor within' each person, which if motivated and supported, can lead to improved health outcomes and better quality of life. The challenge for health professionals is to recognise this concept and learn how to identify and support the 'doctor within' each person with diabetes they have the privilege of caring for.

Chapter 1

Introduction and overview of the book

Introduction

The idea for this book grew from a constant flow of telephone and e-mail requests for advice, particularly from rural health professionals, and responding to letters from people with diabetes in a regular column in *Diabetes Conquest*, a magazine for people with diabetes produced by Diabetes Australia.

Diabetes is a complex, multisystem disease that requires lifelong management in a supportive environment where health professionals work collaboratively with each other and people with diabetes to control the metabolic derangements, prevent complications, and achieve quality of life. The incidence and prevalence of diabetes is increasing globally (King and Rewers 1993; Wild *et al.* 2004; International Diabetes Federation (IDF) 2006). Most health professionals are likely to care for people with diabetes, and often find they have to make clinical decisions without expert support, which many find difficult and challenging. Health professional roles are changing, and new models of care and changed scope of practice are evolving to meet the challenge of the diabetes epidemic facing modern society.

Chronic disease care models have evolved over the past few years and most can be adapted to diabetes. Most encompass methods that address the multifactorial nature of diabetes, and, in Australia, some were developed to address government general practice incentive programmes. Chronic care models need to encompass the following key aspects:

- service delivery, which encompasses leadership and management, appropriately qualified and educated practitioners, patient support, care, and education, delivered in an appropriate environment;

- information systems and communication strategies across the care continuum, including databases and follow-up and referral processes;
- evidence-based practice defined in guidelines and standards;
- monitoring and evaluation/audit processes, which include patient feedback; and
- available and accessible community resources.

Aims of the book

The book aims to support theory and evidence with practical suggestions for managing common clinical problems. The recommendations reflect the education and clinical experience of diabetes educators, endocrinologists, dietitians, general practitioners, and other health professionals who encounter such problems on a daily basis and who have learned to synthesise evidence, clinical experience, and intuition into the care they provide for people with diabetes. The book:

- uses case histories and patient and health professional questions to illustrate diabetes management problems commonly encountered in clinical practice;
- suggests management strategies from the perspective of a range of relevant health professionals who each outline what they see as the key management issues in the case presented and the care they would recommend for the individual. The range of health professionals providing comments about each case reflects diabetes multidisciplinary team care, which is current diabetes best practice;
- cites evidence for the suggested care where possible, but some advice is based on experience; and
- identifies key points that will help health professionals apply the information to other patients with similar problems.

Each chapter commences with a brief introduction to the issues raised by the case studies and questions to provide some background information and context for the management suggested. A list of references and recommended reading can be found at the end of each chapter.

The major focus of the book is on health professionals' recommendations for managing the clinical problems and questions raised in the case histories, which are presented as they were originally received from the person making the referral. Identifying the issues is a key aspect of clinical decision-making. Most cases include comments from a diabetes educator. Others include suggestions from a diabetes specialist, a GP, dietitian, podiatrist and psychologist.

The cases are presented in relevant chapters to ensure that the information is logically presented and easy to locate. These themes include:

- diagnosing diabetes
- managing medicines
- complications
- hyperglycaemia
- complementary therapies
- gestational diabetes
- education and counselling.

It is impossible to discuss every problem that health professionals are likely to encounter. By selecting common problems and suggesting texts where more information can be obtained, the authors hope that health professionals can reflect on the issues raised and the suggested management strategies, and be able to apply the information to other similar cases and settings.

The book reflects the need to blend art and science to arrive at an holistic care plan where the person with diabetes plays a central role in his or her care. *Holistic care* is used to encompass the interconnectedness of the individual with the self (spirituality) and his or her environment, which includes health professionals, and the practical and personal components of a person's life as well as mind, body, and spirit. *Practical* refers to seeking the best management options available to the individual and using a quality use of medicines framework (Department of Health and Aging 2002) to help individuals take stock of – and find meaning in – their lives.

The personal aspects concern the demands that diabetes care places on the individual, his or her responsibility for preventive health care and self-care behaviours (Ventegodt *et al.* 2003a and b). To achieve holistic care, health professionals need to:

- be familiar with a range of management options;
- enter a therapeutic relationship with the individual;
- be effective listeners;
- respect the individual's choice; and
- be reflective practitioners.

In interpreting the information provided by the health professionals in this book, it is important to recognise that 'managing diabetes' is a difficult, lifelong balancing act. The United Kingdom Prospective Diabetes Study (UKPDS) (1998) showed that controlling blood glucose and blood pressure reduced the likelihood of developing microvascular and macrovascular complications, but that maintaining good control in the long term was very difficult. It is important to focus on how guidelines and targets apply to the particular individual at a particular point in time. It is also essential to consider the individual's physical, psychological, spiritual, and social life and environment to achieve life balance and so good metabolic control. The emphasis of care should be on achieving life balance, which is essential to achieving metabolic balance (control). Metabolic control is more likely to occur if life balance (integration and transformation) occurs.

References

Department of Health and Aging (2002) National Strategy for Quality Use of Medicines (www.health.gov.au/internet/wcms/publishing.nsf/Content/nmp-quality.htm).

King H, Rewers M (1993) Global estimates for prevalence of diabetes mellitus and impaired glucose tolerance in adults. WHO Ad Hoc Diabetes Reporting Group. *Diabetes Care* 16(1): 157–177.

United Kingdom Prospective Diabetes Study (UKPDS) 38 (1998) Tight blood pressure control and risk of macrovascular and microvascular complications in type 2 diabetes. *British Medical Journal* 317: 703–713.

Ventegodt S, Anderson N, Merrick J (2003a) Holistic medicine: scientific challenges. *The Scientific World Journal* 3: 1108–1116.

Ventegodt S, Anderson N, Merrick J (2003b) Holistic medicine: the holistic process theory of healing. *The Scientific World Journal* 3: 1138–1146.

Wild S, Roglic G, Green A *et al.* (2004) Global prevalence of diabetes. *Diabetes Care* 27(5): 1047–1053.

Chapter 2

Presentation, diagnosis and classification of diabetes

Key points

- The prevalence of diabetes is increasing globally and is linked to obesity.
- Early diagnosis is important to improve health outcomes.
- Type 2 diabetes is a slow progressive disease, complications are often present at diagnosis, and the symptoms may be vague and attributed to other causes.
- Type 1 diabetes occurs less frequently than type 2 and usually occurs in young people, but it also occurs in older people.
- Gestational diabetes increases the risk of type 2 diabetes.

Introduction

Normal glucose homeostasis depends on hormones, especially insulin and glucagon, tissue sensitivity to insulin, psychological balance, the amount and type of food consumed, nutritional status, and physical activity. Insulin is secreted directly into the portal vein and has a number of actions, including effects on:

- vascular function – insulin deficiency contributes to stiffening and lack of resilience in blood vessel walls and vasodilation in small blood vessels;
- platelets, by inhibiting platelet aggregation;
- the nervous system, including regulating autonomic tone and acting on brain receptors to stimulate sympathetic cardiovascular activity, which assists in blood pressure regulation; and
- electrolyte balance.

In addition, insulin

- promotes glucose uptake in insulin sensitive tissues (muscle and fat);
- inhibits hepatic glucose output;
- promotes glycogen synthesis; and
- stimulates lipolysis protein synthesis to deliver fatty acids and amino acids to muscle and liver for gluconeogenesis.

Rising plasma glucose largely stimulates insulin secretion. Insulin release occurs in two phases:

(1) The first occurs within 10 minutes of the glucose load entering the bloodstream. It reduces hepatic glucose output and is critical to blood glucose balance, because 25–50% of the glucose load is taken up by the liver to be stored as glycogen, which reduces the postprandial blood glucose rise and stores glucose for use in the fasting state and during hypoglycaemia. The first phase response is absent or reduced in type 2 diabetes.
(2) The second phase occurs within 2–4 hours and facilitates glucose entry into the tissues. About 80% of the remaining glucose load is distributed to muscle and 10–25% to adipose tissue. Significantly, insulin resistance is common in type 2 diabetes, so glucose uptake is reduced and the blood glucose levels remain high.

Diabetes mellitus

Diabetes mellitus occurs when carbohydrate, protein and fat metabolism are disturbed due to insulin resistance (type 2 diabetes) or insulin deficiency (type 1 diabetes). As a result, glucose cannot be used for energy and accumulates in the blood, leading to hyperglycaemia and glycosuria. In the longer term, fat and protein stores are mobilised as substrates for gluconeogenesis in the liver. Weight loss and ketone production occurs due to mobilisation of the fat stores, and protein breakdown leads to loss of muscle mass and can affect hormone production and wound healing. Ketone bodies accumulate in the absence of insulin and predispose individuals with type 1 diabetics to ketoacidosis. People with type 2 diabetes are more likely to develop hyperosmolar states, but may become ketotic during severe illness (see Chapter 6).

The main types of diabetes

The main types of diabetes are:

- type 1 diabetes
- type 2 diabetes mellitus
- impaired glucose homeostasis
- gestational diabetes mellitus (GDM).

Type 1 diabetes results from absolute insulin lack. Type 1 is divided into two classes:

- *autoimmune*, where the beta cells are destroyed and autoantibodies can be detected in the blood; and
- *idiopathic* due to unknown causes.

Idiopathic type 1 diabetes is more common in people of Asian descent and autoantibodies are not present in the blood (Tenolouris 2006). These people may present with significant insulinopenia and keto-acidosis. People with type 1 diabetes have an inherited predisposition to diabetes that is triggered by an environmental factor. Suggested causal factors include viruses such as mumps, rubella, Coxsackie B, cytomegalovirus, retrovirus, Epstein–Barr virus, and dietary factors such as cow's milk protein and nitrosamines, which trigger an immune response and set up a chain of slow destruction of the beta cells. Once most of the beta cells are destroyed, symptoms develop rapidly. Sometimes a 'honeymoon' phase occurs once treatment commences and lasts for up to 12 months when small doses of insulin may be required.

Type 2 diabetes mellitus is a heterogenous condition due to both genetic and environmental factors that may be due to defects in insulin secretion or insulin action (insulin resistance and impaired glucose tolerance). Type 2 manifests when both states are present but may take years to manifest. Many people with type 2 diabetes are overweight but it also occurs in lean, often older people, who may in fact have type 1 diabetes or latent autoimmune diabetes in adults (LADA). Testing for glutamic acid decarboxylase (GAD) antibodies helps make the diagnosis.

Significantly, symptoms are often vague, attributed to other causes and to increasing age, and the diagnosis can be delayed. Persistent hyperglycaemia is associated with the early onset of complications: 54% have complications at diagnosis (Colagiuri *et al.* 2002). Infection, which predisposes the individual to hyperosmolar states, occurs in > 13% of respiratory infections occurring in aged care facilities. Active screening is essential to detect diabetes early and address the metabolic defects that lead to hyperglycaemia, including prolonged stress, and disruptive or non-supportive family dynamics (Davis and Renda 2006).

Progressive beta cell destruction also occurs in type 2 diabetes resulting in a 50% decline in insulin production every 5 years (United Kingdom Prospective Diabetes Study (UKPDS) 1998). People need to be educated about the progressive nature of type 2 diabetes to reduce guilt and anxiety about the need for insulin injections and help them understand the need to adhere to the management recommendations. Terms such as 'mild' diabetes give people a false sense of security.

Impaired glucose homeostasis is part of the metabolic syndrome and is an intermediate stage between normal glucose homeostasis and diabetes. It represents a significant risk of cardiovascular disease. Approximately 3% of people with impaired glucose homeostasis progress to diabetes per year.

Gestational diabetes mellitus (GDM) occurs during pregnancy, usually after 28 weeks (see Chapter 10). Women who develop GDM are at risk of developing type 2 diabetes in later life and regular screening to detect diabetes after delivery is recommended (see Chapter 10).

Other specific types of diabetes include diabetes-associated conditions, such as:

- endocrine disorders, e.g. Cushing's disease and acromegaly; and
- medicine- or chemical-induced diabetes (Expert Committee on the Diagnosis and Classification of Diabetes Mellitus 1997).

Prevalence of diabetes

The prevalence of diabetes is high in all ages and both genders, and is increasing globally. However, modern treatment methods mean that people can live long productive lives if:

- the diabetes is effectively managed;
- the individual is involved in his or her own care;
- the individual undertakes appropriate self-care behaviours.

The high prevalence of diabetes alone represents significant direct health costs associated with screening and diagnosis, preventive education and counselling programmes, and managing the disease and its short and long-term complications. Indirect costs include pain, suffering, and the effects of diabetes on the individual's physical and psychological well-being that profoundly affect his or her quality of life.

There is a higher prevalence in older people, who are often diagnosed when they become ill. Regular screening of at-risk individuals can identify glucose intolerance earlier and enable appropriate preventive management strategies to be implemented. Compared with their peers, older people self-report depressive symptoms and are at increased risk of type 2 diabetes. The risk of developing diabetes is independent of other diabetes risk factors (Carnethon 2007). Screening for existing diabetes complications is an important aspect of care, especially given that more than 20% of newly diagnosed people have established complications at diagnosis (National Health and Medical Research Council 1992). In addition, the level of glycaemia at presentation is directly associated with the earlier development of complications (Colagiuri *et al.* 2002).

The diagnosis can be difficult in lean older people. Significantly, autoimmune factors and beta cell destruction can occur in a subset of older people with diabetes, who may have high levels of islet-cell and GAD antibodies, which are markers of autoimmune beta cell destruction and possibly type 1 diabetes. Table 2.1 shows the diabetes diagnostic criteria, Table 2.2 outlines some guidelines for assessing the adequacy of diabetes control, and Table 2.3 indicates diabetes management targets.

Type 1 diabetes in children and young people

More often than not, images of diabetes held by the general public and health professionals are very emotive and conjure up young children injecting insulin with large syringes. Certainly, the diagnosis of type 1 diabetes is more likely to occur during childhood. However, with the

Table 2.1 Fasting plasma glucose is used to diagnose diabetes using World Health Organization criteria (1999). Random plasma glucose or oral glucose tolerance tests are sometimes used. Venous plasma glucose values are also shown. Glucose in capillary blood is about 10–15% higher than venous blood.

Stage	Fasting plasma glucose	Random plasma glucose	Oral glucose tolerance test (OGTT)
Normal	< 6.1 mmol/L		2-hour plasma glucose > 7.8 mmol/L
Impaired glucose tolerance	Impaired fasting glucose: fasting glucose ≥ 6.1 and < 7.0 mmol/L		Impaired glucose tolerance: 2-hour plasma glucose ≥ 7.8 and < 11.1 mmol/L
Diabetes	≥ 7.0 mmol/L	11.1 mmol/L and symptoms	2-hour plasma glucose > 11.1 mmol/L

Table 2.2 Guidelines for assessing metabolic control in people with diabetes.

Haemoglobin A$_{1c}$ (%)*	Glucose (mmol/L)		Level of control
	Fasting	Two hours after food	
4.0–6.0	4	7	Excellent†
6.1–7.4	7	9	Upper limit of normal
7.5–9.4	10	14.5	Unacceptable
> 9.5	14	20	Unacceptable

* When interpreting HbA$_{1c}$ the total clinical picture and history should be considered. False low A$_{1c}$ can occur with anaemia, haemoglobinopathies such as HbS, HbC and HbA, which are found in some ethnic groups, chronic blood loss, haemoptysis, and active haemorrhage. False highs can occur in the presence of chronic alcohol abuse, fetal Hb, and hyperbilirubinaemia.
† May indicate frequent hypoglycaemia.

Table 2.3 Management targets for people with diabetes.

Blood glucose	Fasting 4–6 mmol/L
HbA$_{1c}$	≤ 7%
Cholesterol	< 4.0 mmol/L
Cholesterol LDL	< 2.5 mmol/L
Cholesterol HDL	> 1.0 mmol/L
Triglycerides	> 1.5 mmol/L
Blood pressure	> 130/80 mm Hg
BMI	< 25 kg/m², where possible
Urinary albumin excretion	> 20 μ/min timed overnight collection
	< 20 mg/L spot collection
	< 3.5 mg/mmol (women)
	< 2.5 mg/mmol (men)
Cigarette consumption*	Avoid smoking
Alcohol intake	≤ 4 standard drinks (40 g)/day (men)†
	≤ 2 standard drinks (20 g)/day (women)†
Physical activity	At least 30 minutes of walking (or equivalent) preferably 5 days/week to a total of ≥ 150 minutes/week

* Includes pipe tobacco and cigars.
† Alcohol recommendations are based on the Australian Alcohol Guidelines (2006).
Based on the National Health and Medical Research Council (NHMRC) *Evidence-based Guidelines for the Management of Type 2 Diabetes* (2005).

recognition of latent autoimmune diabetes in adulthood (LADA) an increasing number of adults are being diagnosed with type 1 diabetes.

The incidence of type 1 diabetes in children is increasing worldwide, as is the incidence of type 2 diabetes in this age group, which could even surpass type 1 diabetes in terms of numbers. In 2003, the estimated world child population (0–14) was 1.8 billion, 0.024% with diabetes. This equates to 430 000 children in the world with diabetes and 65 000 new cases diagnosed each year (International Diabetes Federation (IDF) 2006). In the Australian state of Victoria, an average 9.3% increase in the incidence of type 1 diabetes was identified each year between 1999 and 2002 in children under the age of 15 years (Chong *et al.* 2007).

There is little argument among health professionals that the ongoing management and support of young people with diabetes can be complex and demanding. Education and support are not only directed towards the patient – they also involve parents, step-parents or other partners, and often large and complicated blended families. Ongoing diabetes management and support need to address schooling, sport, puberty, sexual activity, driving, drug taking and other risk behaviours.

Diagnosing type 1 diabetes in children is based on blood glucose measurement and the presence (or absence) of symptoms and includes:

- elevated blood glucose level (> 11.1 mmol/L random or 7.0 mmol/L fasting) and symptoms of polyuria, polydipsia, blurred vision, weight loss, glycosuria, and ketonuria;
- diabetic ketoacidosis (DKA) in severe presentations (see Chapter 6); and
- oral glucose tolerance test – only required if symptoms are absent or mild and an elevated blood glucose level occurs under other coexisting stressful situations such as acute infection, trauma, or circulatory stress (Craig *et al.* 2006).

Approximately 1 in 3 children will present with DKA at diagnosis of type 1 diabetes. Significantly, expert care at the time of diagnosis affects re-hospitalisation rates, level of metabolic control, and psychological adjustment/maladjustment (Silink 1996). Understanding the normal stages of childhood and adolescent development and how diabetes can affect these stages is imperative. Initial management and ongoing care and support need to be conscious, systematic, and multidisciplinary. Failure to achieve sound self-management (patient and family actively involved in 'self-management') will lead to impaired growth, delayed puberty, and long-term diabetes complications. Sudden poor glycaemic control after a period of blood glucose stability can result from a variety of causes, including:

- the end of the 'honeymoon' period
- puberty
- family conflict, stress, and breakdown
- stressors at school
- omitting insulin for reasons such as:
  - being tired of having diabetes
  - not wishing to be different anymore
  - seeking attention
  - body image disturbance where insulin is often omitted to reduce weight
- other medical conditions such as hypothyroidism and coeliac disease
- illicit drug taking
- sexual abuse.

Families often talk about the 'costs' of diabetes. The costs of diabetes can include monetary and other less tangible but equally important costs such as the:

- financial burden of diabetes equipment, particular insulin pumps;
- costs associated with stressors placed on the family relationships and roles;
- cost of having nearly all aspects of family life needing to be 'diabetes-friendly,' for example sleepovers, babysitters, and holidays;
- loss of spontaneity from the family unit; and
- parents' fear of failing in their role as diabetes managers.

The key objectives of diabetes education for children and young people and their families are no different from that of adults diagnosed with type 1, type 2 or gestational diabetes. Diabetes education ultimately consists of providing the knowledge, skills and tools the child and family need to be empowered to self-manage. Traditional models of care for newly diagnosed children and young people are changing. Where possible, there is a trend towards providing more education within an ambulatory setting rather than prolonging a hospital admission.

Consensus guidelines identify that 'survival skills education' should occur in 1- to 2-hourly sessions over a 4- to 5-week period (inpatient and increasingly now as an outpatient) or within 2–3 weeks following diagnosis. Ongoing education should occur within the first 12 months of diagnosis. Education sessions should use a variety of strategies lasting 1–2 hours in duration over 8–16 sessions. Longer term, there should be at least one annual education review (Silink 1996). No matter how or where education is delivered, it will be intense and complex, requiring the team to possess excellent communication skills, compassion, sensitivity, humour, and in depth knowledge of child-hood diabetes (Silverstein *et al.* 2005).

The age of the child and their level of maturity determine the degree of self-management they are able to undertake. Infants, toddlers, and early school-aged children usually require the parents and other adults to be the primary self-manager. School-aged children over the age of eight generally assume more of the daily diabetes tasks. Often insulin pumps are introduced to this age group. Parents of young people can be tempted to hand over total diabetes self-management. However, it is recommended that parents maintain some degree of guidance and supervision. Adolescence is often a time where the diabetes team can assist in renegotiating the roles and responsibilities of each family member and the young person with diabetes to reduce conflict and poor glycaemic outcomes during what can be a difficult time for everybody.

Blood glucose targets are also determined by age (Table 2.4). For example, children under the age of six often have very unpredictable food intake and levels of physical activity. Hypoglycaemia can be common. Young children are often unable to communicate their hypoglycaemia symptoms and all parents fear cognitive impairment, even brain damage resulting from severe hypoglycaemia. HbA_{1c} targets are thus different for children of different ages (Silverstein *et al.* 2005).

Using insulin pumps or new basal and bolus analogue insulins may achieve HbA_{1c} targets < 7.0%, which is promoted for adults with diabetes. Such targets should only be strived for in children if the number and degree of hypoglycaemic episodes can be minimised. However, basal insulins such as glargine and determir have not been approved for use in children younger than 6 years in Australia. Other adult management strategies such as the Dose Adjustment for Normal Eating (DAFNE) programme are not available to individuals with type 1 diabetes younger than 18 years.

An understanding of dietary requirements is imperative and includes understanding calorie restriction in an overweight child

Table 2.4 Target HbA_{1c} levels according to age range in children and young people.

Age group	HbA_{1c} target
< 6 years	7.5–8.5%
6–12 years	8.0%
13–19 years	< 7.5%

with type 1 diabetes, and increased caloric requirements during puberty. Strategies to cope with eating out and feeling part of a group of friends are very important for a child or teenager. Children with and without diabetes should all perform 30–60 minutes of physical activity daily. Children with diabetes need to know how to reduce their risk of hypoglycaemia and if it does occur, how to treat low blood glucose levels effectively. Blood testing times and frequency should be well established and the benefits of testing be promoted in terms of self-management. They should be able to undertake activities such as sport, eating fast food occasionally, and sleepovers with their friends. Sick day management plans are required not only for home, but for day care and schools.

In terms of long-term diabetes complications, the following screening should occur:

- annual screening for microalbuminuria once the child is over the age of 10 and/or has had diabetes for 5 years;
- for prepubertal children, a fasting lipid profile performed on all children over the age of 2 years at the time of diagnosis to be repeated once the child reaches 12 years of age;
- ophthalmologic examination in children over the age of 10 years who have had diabetes for at least 3 years; and
- annual foot examination once puberty commences (Silverstein *et al.* 2005).

CASE DISCUSSION

Mrs TP

Mrs TP was referred to a tertiary diabetes clinic by a rural GP
Please advise about this 50-year-old female with supposed type 1 diabetes, which she has had for some years.

She is on Protaphane 12 units nocte.

Her blood glucose ranges between 3 and 6 mmol/L fasting, rising to about 8.2 mmol/L post-food.

HbA_{1c} usually 7.4%.

She is having hypos (hypo unawareness) at lunchtime, but increased her own morning NovoRapid because she thought her HbA_{1c} was high. Basically she cannot understand the difference between her blood glucose tests and HbA_{1c}.

Her old notes show no GAD antibodies but she did initially present in a comatose state following a three-stone weight loss.

What else should I do for this woman?

Diabetes educator

Three key issues need to be addressed:

(1) What type of diabetes does Mrs TP have?
(2) How can the frequency of hypoglycaemic episodes be reduced to enable her to recognise symptoms again?
(3) Mrs TP should stop driving until her hypoglycaemia unawareness resolves.

Mrs TP's history is relatively common in tertiary diabetes centres but may be uncommon in general practice. The type of diabetes Mrs TP has is unclear. She may have type 1 diabetes. Up to 80% of people with type 1 diabetes exhibit either GAD or IA_2 antibodies, which means that 20% do not have such antibodies but may still have type 1 diabetes. Measuring her C-peptide would demonstrate how much insulin her pancreas produces. A normal or raised C-peptide level suggests type 2 diabetes, while a low level suggests type 1 diabetes. Measuring her IA_2 antibodies would also be useful because people with type 1 diabetes can be positive for IA_2 and not GAD antibodies. Mrs TP was diagnosed with a three-stone weight loss, which suggests type 1 diabetes. Often people with type 2 diabetes present with weight gain rather than weight loss.

People with type 1 diabetes are at risk of developing diabetic ketoacidosis (DKA) and this may account for her comatose state on presentation. Alternatively, the coma might have been due to hyperosmolar non-ketonic coma (HONK). There is no mention of ketones or indication of her pH on presentation, which again could suggest the diabetes type. The initial treatment for both DKA and HONK is insulin, which is required permanently in type 1 and often for several weeks or months following recovery from HONK, after which oral hypoglycaemic agents can be slowly introduced once the blood glucose levels are stable. During the recovery period the beta cells start to produce more insulin. If a definitive diagnosis of type 1 diabetes cannot be made, insulin should be slowly withdrawn over a period of weeks and oral agents introduced.

However, if insulin therapy needs to be maintained, Mrs TP's current insulin regimen needs to be revised. Bedtime intermediate-acting insulin has variable effects on the blood glucose. Its peak action can be anywhere from 4–12 hours after administration and last up to 24 hours. The site of administration affects the onset of action and therefore its peak effect. The abdomen is the preferred injection site because the action profile is more predictable.

These are the possible management options:

- Her prescription could be changed from Protaphane to a long-acting basal analogue such as Lantus or Levemir to improve the fasting blood glucose levels, which will in turn contribute to a reduction in HbA_{1c} and reduce the need to increase the breakfast dose of NovoRapid. Hypoglycaemia before lunch is more likely to be due to her bedtime Protaphane than her breakfast NovoRapid dose, which peaks approximately 90 minutes after administration and is almost completely gone by mid-morning.
- If Mrs TP does have type 2 diabetes, combining the basal analogue insulin with an oral agent such as the sustained release metformin (Diabex XR) may be the first step towards eventually ceasing insulin therapy and using oral agents to maintain glycaemic control.
- A three-day period of continuous blood glucose monitoring could help identify when Mrs TP becomes hypoglycaemic – which may occur at times other than when she tests her blood glucose – and identify hypoglycaemic unawareness. Significant hypoglycaemia may mean that Mrs TP should not drive her car until she can recognise hypoglycaemia symptoms and her blood glucose levels are stable, which may impact on her employment and will need to be managed sensitively.

Mrs TP is not the only person to find it difficult to understand the difference between the HbA_{1c} and capillary blood glucose tests. Many health professionals do not know the difference. HbA_{1c} measures the red blood cell exposure to glucose over a 3-month period. However, a number of factors can affect the accuracy of the HbA_{1c} result. For example, an HbA_{1c} of 7.4% could occur due to the daily blood glucose fluctuations between 3 and 8.2 mmol/L that Mrs TP reports. Her fasting blood glucose range is a little too low (4–6 mmol/L would be preferable) and may mean she consumes extra fast-acting carbohydrate to correct hypoglycaemia, which in turn could cause a postprandial glucose excursion. Although the fasting blood glucose levels contribute to an HbA_{1c} under 7%, high postprandial readings account for most of the rise in HbA_{1c}.

In addition, a number of other medical conditions directly affect the lifespan of red blood cells and consequently the accuracy of the HbA_{1c}. Schneider (2006) described 700 different variables that could possibly affect the HbA_{1c}. Despite these limitations, the HbA_{1c} is a valuable indicator of metabolic control. However, it should be interpreted considering the clinical picture and the day-to-day capillary blood glucose results. The accuracy of Mrs TP's blood glucose testing technique should be checked and it is important to ensure that:

- her meter is calibrated correctly;
- the strips/electrodes are within the expiry date;
- her technique is correct; and
- when she tests in relation to food is recorded.

Generally, the accepted time to measure blood glucose after meals is 2 hours after eating. Testing earlier measures the post absorptive state rather than postprandial. If Mrs TP tests 30 minutes after eating, her results will be falsely raised and will not be a true indication of her postprandial glycaemic control. In summary, I suggest the following.

- Measure her IA_2 antibodies and C-peptide to determine whether she has type 1 or type 2 diabetes.
- Review her medical notes at the time of diagnosis to ascertain:
  - whether ketones were present at diagnosis
  - the pH at the time.
- Check her blood glucose meter and testing technique.
- Elicit more information about when she tests her blood glucose, administers her insulin, and how she manages hypoglycaemia.
- Check her injection sites.
- Explore the feasibility of 72 hours of continuous blood glucose monitoring to identify when and how often her blood glucose levels drop below 3.5 mmol/L without accompanying symptoms.
- If the review of her medical record at the time of diagnosis and the results of the recommended blood test indicate she has type 2 diabetes, start to gradually wean her off insulin and commence oral hypoglycaemic agents, in particular, metformin.

Dietitian

Mrs TP's story raises several issues: does she really need insulin?

I would like more information about how she makes decisions about her NovoRapid doses. She is on a relatively small basal insulin dose and has an exceptionally good blood glucose range, possibly too low. I would aim to increase the range to 4–7 mmol/L. Is she using appropriate NovoRapid doses and an algorithm to adjust the doses?

I would determine her lifestyle, weight and activity level to determine whether her insulin sensitivity could be improved and insulin resistance reduced. The consistency of her carbohydrate intake needs to be checked and she may need to be educated about carbohydrate counting, glycaemic index (GI) and mixed meals.

Despite her tight control (HbA$_{1c}$ 7.4%) Mrs TP may need more education about her meals and blood glucose testing especially the difference between pre- and postprandial test results.

I would take the opportunity to review her dietary intake by taking a detailed diet history, which could be compared with accepted nutritional recommendations (50–55% carbohydrate, 30–35% saturated fat, 10–15% protein) (Canadian Diabetes Association 2003; American Diabetes Association 2004; Diabetes Nutrition Study Group 2004). I would use a plate model or food pyramid to demonstrate a balanced diet pictorially. In addition, I would promote physical activity and aim to achieve a body mass index (BMI)/waist circumference within normal limits.

Endocrinologist

As well as the comments above, several further points could be addressed.

First, the disparity of the HbA$_{1c}$ with capillary glucoses might be clarified by measuring serum fructosamine, which represents a glycosylated component of serum proteins, reflecting the average blood glucose over the previous 2–3 weeks while not being influenced by red blood cell turnover or the level of haemoglobin variants. The HbA$_{1c}$ could also be measured by an affinity method, which is less affected by haemoglobin variants, and combined with haemoglobin electrophoresis to explore the presence of such variants. Renal function should be measured, because carbamylated haemoglobin, which is raised according to the severity of renal impairment, can cross-react in some HbA$_{1c}$ assays. It is now clear that some patients glycosylate their own tissues at a higher-than-normal rate for the same average glucose levels.

Second, it needs to be kept in mind that we now know that hypoglycaemic unawareness in a percentage of patients can be reversed, and is secondary to the hypoglycaemia itself 'stunning' the autonomic nervous system. The stunning impairs the development of the typical 'adrenergic' symptoms characteristic of hypoglycaemia. The way to confirm whether this process is occurring is to concentrate on eliminating hypoglycaemia, even if metabolic control is temporarily poor, until the warning signs return. The doses of NovoRapid insulin were not specified, but reducing the breakfast dose would be critical in this patient to eliminate the lunchtime hypoglycaemia. Her target glucose should be 5–8 mmol/L before meals and any glucose levels less than 4 more than occasionally would trigger a dose readjustment.

Diabetes educator 2

While accepting the previous comments, I suggest that Mrs TP's insulin sensitivity is not in question since her control is very good. Nor does insulin resistance appear to be a problem given her HbA_{1c} and capillary blood glucose range. In addition to the issues already raised, her menopausal status needs to be evaluated. Menopause occurs at around 51 years of age and Mrs TP is 51, so she is likely to be peri- or postmenopausal and her changing hormone status could affect her blood glucose levels.

Oestrogen production has individual effects on blood glucose, which can often be more variable and contribute to symptoms such as mood changes, fatigue and hot flushes that can be mistaken for hypoglycaemia. Menopausal symptoms often occur at night and compromise sleep. Blood glucose testing, including at the time she experiences the symptoms, will help determine the cause. If the symptoms are due to the menopause, Mrs TP may be unnecessarily consuming extra calories that can compromise her control.

Her medicines may need to be reviewed and possibly adjusted. The need for other medicines – such as lipid-lowering agents, antihypertensive agents and low-dose aspirin – should be assessed and her weight monitored, because it is common for women to gain weight after menopause.

Women who are obese at the time of menopause are also at greater risk of developing breast cancer due to higher levels of oestrogen as a result of excess abdominal fat (Bernstein 2002). If she smokes she should be counselled to stop. She should discuss menopausal symptom management with her doctor. Short-term hormone replacement therapy (HRT) may be indicated, but the benefits need to be weighed against the risk of breast cancer. If HRT is indicted, the lowest effective dose should be used for the shortest possible time (Khoo and Mahesh 2005). Mrs TP might like to consider complementary therapies such as Dong Quai, red clover and black cohosh, which help relieve symptoms for some but not all women. Mrs TP may be at increased risk of osteoporosis after menopause and her diet and activity may need to be revised.

I would also take the opportunity to check when she last had a pap smear, mammogram and general health check and refer her for the relevant investigations if necessary. Bone density studies might be useful, particularly if she smokes.

Sexual dysfunction in women is a prevalent problem and needs to be considered with Mrs TP. In most cases, neither the woman nor her health professionals discuss the issue (Ohl 2007). Female dysfunction is more often psychogenic in origin than male sexual dysfunction. However, it has been linked to medical conditions such as hypertension and antihypertensive medications (Burchardt *et al.* 2002), diabetes (Enzlin *et al.* 2002), and coronary artery diseases (Salonia *et al.* 2002). It appears the vascular complications that cause male erectile dysfunction are associated with sexual dysfunction in women, especially at the arousal stage.

In addition, the hypoglycaemia could be associated with sexual activity. Taking a careful sexual history could help identify whether Mrs TP is experiencing any sexual difficulties or has any other stressors, or psychological issues that could be affecting her blood glucose levels and quality of life. Specific management would depend on the findings. The PLISST model (permission, limited information, specific suggestions, and intensive therapy) (Annon 1976; Dunning 1993) is a useful framework for providing sexual counselling and can help health professionals identify their level of competence to do so.

CASE DISCUSSION

Mrs TZ

Mrs TZ was referred by a podiatrist
Mrs TZ is a 50-year-old woman with type 1 (she assures me this is a correct diagnosis) and she has been diagnosed for some years. She is currently on 12 units nocte Protaphane and 6 units TDS NovoRapid.

She has recently been experiencing hypos or more hypo unawareness. Around lunchtime, her blood glucose is usually between 3 and 6 mmol/L and her postprandial test is no higher than 8.2 mmol/L. She recently increased her morning dose of NovoRapid.

Her hypos are happening at about 1.8–1.4 mmol. She sometimes gets blurred vision, and sweating.

Mrs TZ works full-time in an office, and although her colleagues know she has diabetes, during her last episode, her boss left her alone, a little scary for both I think, but her main concern is she may hypo when she is driving.

I wonder whether she is type 2 late onset? I would appreciate your advice, thanks.

Diabetes educator

My immediate response would be to address the hypoglycaemia. Because the hypoglycaemia occurs before lunch I would reduce her breakfast NovoRapid by 2 units, initially bearing in mind that is approximately 30% of her dose. People are taught to adjust their insulin in 1- to 2-unit increments up to 4 units. I would review her hypoglycaemia management to ensure that she takes simple (fast-acting) carbohydrate, for example 5–7 jellybeans or 100 ml of Lucozade or lemonade at the first sign of a hypo and follows with some complex (slow-acting) carbohydrate. In Mrs TZ's case, this could be her lunch, ensuring that it includes complex carbohydrate. She should be advised to retest her blood glucose after 30 minutes to make sure her blood glucose is rising. If the symptoms of hypogly-caemia have not resolved after 10 minutes, she should eat another 15 g of fast-acting carbohydrate.

Blurred vision and sweating are common hypoglycaemic symptoms. Other symptoms include trembling, weakness, hunger and nervousness. These symptoms vary among people with diabetes. Most people recognise their symptoms, but Mrs TZ is experiencing hypoglycaemic unawareness, which can be exacerbated by the frequent episodes of hypoglycaemia and the duration of diabetes. Hypoglycaemic unawareness means that people do not recognise the early symptoms so they progress and the brain does not get enough glucose. Confusion, drowsiness and changes in behaviour followed by coma and possibly seizure occur. This is a very serious situation. It requires another party to manage the hypoglycaemia and assist with resuscitation. This includes protecting the airway and injecting glucagon if it is available or calling an ambulance. Educating and supporting the family is very important.

Mrs TZ should be referred to her general practitioner to determine whether she has type 1 or type 2 diabetes (see case discussion Mrs TP). Meanwhile, the diabetes educator should assess Mrs TZ's diabetes self-management, the accuracy of her blood glucose meter through quality control testing, ensuring the blood glucose strips are in date, checking her testing technique, testing and recording frequency and accuracy by downloading the blood glucose test record stored in the meter memory. All of these steps help eliminate user error, which is often unintentional.

Review insulin administration by checking:

- the insulin delivery device;
- Mrs TZ's technique;
- injection sites;
- that she is not injecting into the same area all the time, which can cause hypertrophy and interfere with insulin absorption; and
- the dosing accuracy of her insulin pen (dial up 20 units and deliver the dose into the plastic pen needle cap. If the level of insulin in the cap is to the bottom of the flange, the dose is accurate).

Asking Mrs TZ how she adjusts her insulin will help determine whether she adjusts her dose correctly. I suggest she needs more education about insulin action because she increased her insulin dose at breakfast despite becoming hypoglycaemic around lunchtime, which suggests the pre-breakfast dose should be reduced.

I would refer her to a dietitian for a dietary review and to ensure she has adequate carbohydrate with her breakfast. She may in fact omit breakfast. I would also discuss exercise with her, because it could be another cause of her hypoglycaemia. Some people can experience hypoglycaemia many hours after exercise.

Mrs TZ's boss knows she has diabetes and expects her to be responsible for her diabetes care at work. He and other employees need to be able to manage hypoglycaemia, but her employment may be jeopardised if she does not appropriately monitor her diabetes and have regular medical reviews. People with diabetes cannot be (nor do they want to be) in the company of another person 24 hours a day.

Sensible blood glucose monitoring and adherence to her diet will reduce the risk of hypoglycaemia and improve her safety at work as well as when she is driving. It is essential she tests her blood glucose before driving to ensure it is at a safe level (for example > 5.0 mmol/L) and has simple carbohydrate with her at all times. Mrs TZ is on insulin and is required to have an annual fitness to drive assessment by the Motor Traffic Authority before her driver's license is renewed. The review includes a medical check-up, history of hypoglycaemia, vision check and diabetes assessment to ensure she is safe to drive and does not put herself or others on the road at risk.

General practitioner

Many patients inform the GP that they have type 1 and are usually correct if they use that term. However, many people often describe their diagnosis as insulin-requiring when the diagnosis may be less straightforward. A good history will often give the diagnosis. Mrs TZ has had her diabetes for many years, and her particular pattern of insulin use with relatively small doses suggests type 1 but other findings such as body mass index (BMI), duration of diabetes before commencing insulin, and initial presentation would help establish the diagnosis.

Late onset type 1 refers to a situation where people develop type 1 diabetes at a much older age than usually expected. These patients often have a normal BMI; the so-called lean diabetic. A significant proportion of older people develop late onset type 1 diabetes (LADA), possibly approximately 20% of patients diagnosed with type 2 diabetes.

Patients with a normal BMI or those who require increasing doses of medication very quickly should be tested for anti-GAD antibodies. It is important to identify this group of patients, because they will require insulin much earlier than patients with type 2. They are also at risk of ketoacidosis. Late-onset type 2 diabetes may be confused with the older term 'mature onset diabetes,' which is now called type 2 diabetes.

Hypoglycaemic events can be very frightening, more so when symptoms suddenly occur due to hypoglycaemic unawareness. Patients may become confused or collapse due to the lack of warning and be unable to treat the hypoglycaemia. Unfortunately, as patients are treated more aggressively to prevent complications, the number of hypoglycaemic reactions patients endure is also likely to increase. Hypos in the workplace can be an issue. Regular glucose monitoring during the day, ready access to a quick source of glucose, and regular meal times are important. It is useful for fellow workers to be aware of the risk of hypos so they can help if a severe hypo should occur.

Mrs TZ has also identified a major issue of safety when driving, which is especially important since she has hypo unawareness. Mrs TZ should always check her blood glucose before driving and have ready access to quick-acting glucose in the car.

Current recommendations from the Austroads driver guidelines (Austroads 2006) indicate that if a driver has a 'defined' hypo the driver should be advised not to drive for 6 weeks or until cleared by a specialist. If a hypoglycaemic episode occurs while driving and is the cause of a car accident the driver licensing authority should be notified. A 'defined' hypoglycaemic event relevant to driving is one of sufficient severity to impair perception or motor skills, cause abnormal behaviour or impair consciousness. It is different from mild hypoglycaemic symptoms such as sweating, trembling, hunger, and tingling around the mouth, which are common occurrences in the life of a person with diabetes treated with insulin and some oral hypoglycaemic agents.

The pattern of glucose control is important when adjusting the insulin dose to avoid hypos and to retain good control. There is evidence that the newer long-acting insulins such as Lantus can give the same level of control but with fewer hypos. Education about appropriate insulin self-adjustment during changes in meals or exercise is important for all patients with diabetes. The doses of NovoRapid insulin were not specified, but reduction of the breakfast dose would be critical in this patient, aiming to eliminate the lunchtime hypoglycaemia. Her target glucose should be 5–8 mmol/L before meals and any glucose level under 4 more than occasionally would trigger an insulin dose readjustment.

Endocrinologist

The driving issues are serious in patients having major or 'defined' hypoglycaemic episodes and the Austroads guidelines are an important advance in trying to harmonise the approach in different Australian states and territories. Other countries have similar initiatives and it is important to note that the legal implications vary significantly in different countries and indeed different states and territories within Australia. While the guidelines are very useful, it is critical to be aware of the specific legal requirements in the particular practice location. For example, the requirement for health professionals to notify the relevant driving authorities of concerns varies considerably. The legal protection given to the health professional who might notify authorities or fill in reports also varies within Australia and internationally. The other complication is that, even if there is indemnification, the civil legal system might still allow a health professional to be joined in legal actions with a defendant when damages are sought. In summary, it is critical to be informed, not only about the specific regulations in a practice location, but also the non-regulatory civil legal implications.

CASE DISCUSSION

Mr BE

Mr BE was referred by a nurse working in acute care
Mr BE is a 78-year-old male who had lithotripsy yesterday. He had an incidental random glucose 12.8 BGLs on ward range between 7 and 13. He is not a known diabetic but his GP told him he has borderline diabetes. Both his sisters developed diabetes later in life.

His fasting glucose is 8.5 mmol/L and his fasting lipids are slightly elevated. He is having an HbA$_{1c}$ tomorrow.
Please advise.

General practitioner

Mr BE has diabetes (see Figure 2.1). I would check that this fasting glucose performed was a laboratory result to ensure it was accurate. Blood glucose meters have an error of up to 10% or more if they are not calibrated or outdated strips are used. It is important for people with 'borderline diabetes' to have a glucose tolerance test (GTT)

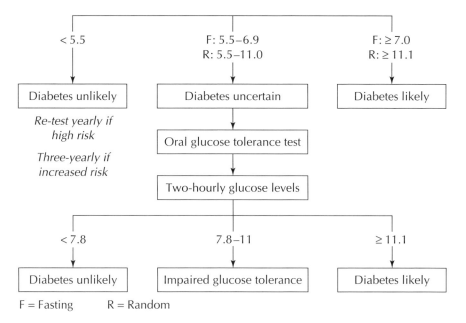

Figure 2.1 Glucose levels in venous plasma (mmol/L).
Source: Diabetes Australia and RACGP Diabetes Management in General Practice 2005–2006

because some people with a fasting glucose between 5.5 and 7.0 mmol/L have diabetes. Mr BE should then have at least a fasting glucose or repeat GTT annually.

It is important to diagnose diabetes early so that you can institute appropriate treatment and prevent complications. Five percent of people with diabetes have complications at diagnosis, which indicates that many people have had diabetes long before they were initially diagnosed. The Australian diabetes, obesity and lifestyle study (AusDiab) (Dunstan *et al.* 2000) demonstrated that for each person with known diabetes there is another one undiagnosed.

The use of terms such as 'borderline diabetes' or 'mild diabetes' is unhelpful and can often lead to people being reassured inappropriately. Diabetes is a serious illness with significant morbidity and mortality. Early diagnosis and management is essential to prevent or appropriately manage long-term complications. People with diabetes have a risk of heart disease equivalent to people in the general population who have already had a myocardial infarct. This risk extends to patients with 'pre-diabetes;' that is those with impaired fasting glucose or impaired glucose tolerance.

It is likely that Mr BE has type 2 diabetes with such a strong family history of diabetes in his sisters. Type 2 diabetes has a stronger genetic link than type 1. The chance of having type 1 diabetes is approximately 8% if one parent has type 1 diabetes. The risk is 25% for type 2 diabetes if a parent has type 2 diabetes.

Endocrinologist

The criteria for diagnosis during a glucose tolerance test assume the test was conducted under conditions recommended by the WHO. This includes not doing the test after recent surgery, where the metabolic response to injury will cause impaired glucose tolerance. Whether lithotripsy is sufficient to explain the current results is not certain, but it would be advisable to repeat the fasting glucose about 6 weeks following the procedure and proceed to oral glucose tolerance test (OGTT) if the fasting plasma glucose is at or above 5.5 mmol/L at that time.

Diabetes educator

Mr BE has a strong family history of diabetes and may have diabetes, but it is difficult to diagnose diabetes accurately in acute situations as the endocrinologist indicated. Stress hyperglycaemia often accompanies critical illness, is usually transient and resolves when the acute situation resolves. The hyperglycaemia is most likely due to the counter-regulatory hormone response, increased sympathetic nervous system activity, increased lipolysis and free fatty acids, and reduced insulin secretion. The hyperglycaemia does need to be managed (aim 4–6 mmol/L) because it is associated with increased morbidity such as impaired white cell function, infection, stroke and myocardial infarction in diabetics and non-diabetics (American Association of Clinical Endocrinologists 2003).

It is important to establish whether Mr BE does have diabetes. Given his age he may already have diabetes complication(s) and new diagnosis is associated with a higher rate of complications in older people and greater mortality (Bethel *et al.* 2007). Older people with newly diagnosed diabetes are twice as likely to have lower leg complications such as pain, cellulitis and gangrene, cardiovascular disease, chronic renal failure and end-stage renal disease, low vision and blindness (Bethel *et al.* 2007). A full complication assessment is warranted.

The HbA_{1c} provides useful information but it is not a diagnostic test. Traditionally, an OGTT is recommended in cases such as

Mr BE. However, recent research suggests non-invasive spectroscopic measurements of advanced glycation end products (AGE) in the skin may be useful, accurate, and less invasive (Maynard 2007). AGE are 'biomarkers of diabetes' and are closely associated with and predictive of diabetes complications especially retinopathy and nephropathy and are more sensitive at diagnosing diabetes than fasting glucose or HbA_{1c}. However, the test is not widely used at present and may not be available where Mr BE is being managed.

Studies such as the Diabetes Prevention Programme (Knowler *et al.* 2002), the Finnish Diabetes Prevention Study (Tuomilehto *et al.* 2001) and the Da Quing study (Pan *et al.* 1997) demonstrate that lifestyle interventions (diet, exercise and weight management) can prevent diabetes. Metformin (Knowler *et al.* 2002) and acarbose (Chiasson *et al.* 2002) may also have a role in prevention. Rosiglitazone may also prevent the onset of type 2 diabetes but is associated with higher risk of myocardial infarction and heart failure (Nissen and Wolski 2007) and may be contraindicated in older people such as Mr BE. Ramipril normalises blood glucose levels but does not reduce the incidence of diabetes (Bosch *et al.* 2006). More recently Schultze *et al.* (2007) demonstrated that high-fibre diets from cereal (but not fruit and vegetables) and insoluble fibre reduce the risk of diabetes. A meta-analysis also indicated high magnesium diets were associated with lower rates of diabetes (Schultze *et al.* 2007).

Mr BE needs advice about lifestyle measures such as high fibre low fat diet, exercise, and regular follow-up. He needs to receive sensitive advice about his diabetes risks and the positive actions he can take to reduce the risk. He should not be told he has mild diabetes under any circumstances (see the next case study). I would provide him with basic advice about reducing his risk of diabetes or controlling his diabetes and refer him to a dietitian and his GP for regular follow-up.

CASE DISCUSSION

Mrs MZE

Mrs MZE was referred by a nurse in a general medical ward
We were discussing diabetes during handover today. One woman who used to have type 2 on tablets has been commenced on insulin so I guess her diabetes is now serious, as she now has type 1.
  She needs education please.

Diabetes educator

Mrs MZE still has type 2 diabetes. Type 2 diabetes is associated with slow progressive destruction of the beta cells and insulin is required in > 50% of people with type 2 diabetes with increasing disease duration. The belief that type 2 diabetes 'will become worse and need insulin and turn into type 1, and therefore more serious disease' is a common misconception among health professionals and people with diabetes. Diabetes is a serious disease regardless of diabetes type and treatment mode.

Her education will involve ascertaining how she feels about starting insulin and explaining why she needs to have insulin. She should be involved in selecting an insulin delivery device and insulin regimen. She will need to know how to:

- manage her insulin;
- administer a dose;
- recognise and treat hypoglycaemia;
- dispose of sharps safely; and
- (eventually) how to adjust her insulin doses.

I would refer her to a dietitian for dietary advice (see Chapters 4 and 9).

CASE DISCUSSION

Jade

Jade was referred to the diabetes management team following admission to the emergency department
Jade, an 11-year-old girl, was admitted via the emergency department with hyperglycaemia, ketonuria and a weight loss of 6 kg over the past 4 weeks. The only history of diabetes in her family is her maternal grandfather with type 2 diabetes. Arterial blood gases indicate that she is ketonic but not in DKA and she was admitted to a medical ward for stabilisation.

Diabetes educator

It appears Jade has type 1 diabetes. Ultimately the diagnosis can be confirmed by measuring her GAD and IA_2 antibodies and C-peptide. Her initial treatment is rehydration, correcting the hyperglycaemia and 'survival skills education'. Following intravenous rehydration and correcting the blood glucose levels using an insulin infusion, education on subcutaneous insulin begins.

Survival skills education involves providing enough information and support for Jade and her family to manage safely at home following discharge (Queensland Health 2002; see Chapter 9). This could occur after 3–5 days of admission. The four areas include:

(1) insulin administration
(2) blood glucose monitoring
(3) basic diet information
(4) hypoglycaemia detection, treatment and prevention.

An understanding and ability for Jade and her family to perform basic activities around these areas are imperative before discharge. The type of education provided by the team needs to be adaptable, personalised and appropriate to Jade's age, maturity and lifestyle. Often a diagnosis of diabetes at this time for the teenager and their family is characterised by confusion, fear, anger, denial, and disbelief. All of these emotions are normal responses to a diagnosis of type 1 diabetes in a child. Everyone in the family needs to be supported and introduced to the diabetes team, which usually includes a medical specialist, diabetes educator, dietitian and psychologist.

Where possible, Jade will be encouraged to undertake as much of her care as possible with the support and supervision of her family. Involving siblings is also important. Managing newly diagnosed children requires an enormous amount of hospital resources. It is important to find the balance between what the patient and family needs to know to get them out of hospital and manage the diabetes over the next few weeks. Young children require families to provide diabetes management and teenagers should not be expected to undertake all their care independently. However, the eventual transition to independent self-management is some years off for Jade and adult involvement is imperative. A recent study demonstrated that mothers' diabetes knowledge directly correlated with variability in insulin injection times and blood glucose parameters. Children whose mothers had better knowledge had less variability in insulin injection times, more frequent blood glucose testing, and lower HbA_{1c} levels (Chisholm *et al.* 2007).

Jade may initially be in a 'honeymoon' period with respect to her insulin requirements. That is, she will still be producing her own insulin for possibly the next 6 months and, therefore, require only a small dose of exogenous insulin. For example, daily or twice daily insulin, basal analogue or a basal and bolus analogue twice daily should be sufficient. It is rare that insulin is required at this stage 4–5 times/day. It is unlikely that an insulin pump would be used initially given the complexity of the system, the sheer volume of information the family needs to learn, and the number of changes to lifestyle for the entire family. The duration of the 'honeymoon' period appears related to a number of factors. On the whole they generally last around 6–7 months. Shorter honeymoon periods appear related to being aged younger than 5 years at diagnosis, presenting in DKA at initial diagnosis, and having a longer duration of symptoms before diagnosis (Abdul-Rasoul *et al.* 2006).

At this time a social worker may also be of help to outline the type of financial supports that could be available to the family to assist them to manage Jade's diabetes. Other issues that need to be addressed include contacting Jade's school to outline the role and expectations of the school, Jade, and her family with respect to managing her diabetes. Blood glucose meters are available free of charge to children with type 1 diabetes in Australia. Many diabetes health professionals encourage people with type 1 diabetes to use meters that also test blood ketone levels, especially during illness. These meters are also useful in emergency departments to enable early diagnosis of ketoacidosis and faster treatment (Nauheim *et al.* 2006).

Often, after parents research diabetes via the internet and books, they realise that severe hypoglycaemia can result in cognitive impairment. Not surprisingly, this can result in great anxiety for parents and may lead to keeping BGLs higher than desired. Such anxiety may or may not be eased when parents are taught to administer glucagon. There is sometimes an expectation that teaching staff at schools should be trained to administer insulin and glucagon. However, the most appropriate response to such requests is to provide school staff with:

- information and skills for basic hypoglycaemia care;
- the knowledge to recognise when an ambulance should be called;
- policies outlining where Jade's insulin should be stored; and
- policies outlining when she is to self-administer.

Following hospital discharge, close ongoing contact and additional education are required. It is well established that ongoing education in the early period following diagnosis and discharge is critical to determining both quality of life and clinical outcomes (International Society for Pediatric and Adolescent Diabetes (ISPAD) 2000). It can be a fine line between creating a relationship of co-dependence with the diabetes team and empowering the patients and their families. A whole additional range of areas need to be addressed including:

- sport with insulin and carbohydrate adjustment
- sick day management
- adjusting insulin doses

- sleepovers and camps
- birthday parties and other festive eating.

However, not all newly diagnosed patients live geographically close to a multidisciplinary paediatric diabetes team, and the diabetes team needs to engage with other health providers to assist these families such as the general practitioner, adult diabetes educator, and paediatrician.

Longer-term issues will include how puberty affects glycaemic control, how to manage diabetes once the 'honeymoon' ends and risk behaviours such as smoking, alcohol and illicit drug taking. When there is no endogenous insulin left, there is often far more variation in blood glucose levels from injected insulin. Therefore, the child is at increased risk of severe hyperglycaemia and DKA. Months after the diagnosis of diabetes, the 'novelty' (if there really was ever a novelty) wears off for the patient and his/her family. They often want their previous life and lifestyle back, where they eat what they want and do what they want without the daily restrictions of type 1 diabetes.

Regular and ongoing involvement by a psychologist is vital. At each clinic visit Jade should have her height and weight plotted on a growth chart, which is an excellent additional marker to her general health and metabolic control (Silverstein *et al.* 2005). Thyroid function and coeliac antibodies should be measured if unexplained weight loss occurs.

Raised HbA_{1c} may indicate more than just suboptimal blood glucose control. Researchers have identified a correlation between the rates of depression and high HbA_{1c} levels (Hood *et al.* 2006). It may also be a 'cry for help' relating to other issues at home (see Chapter 8).

One thing to keep in mind, particularly for teenage girls with type 1 diabetes, is body image. Commencing insulin injections usually leads to an increase in weight. Over-treatment of insulin can cause significant weight gain, even obesity. If Jade experiences frequent hypos, and therefore eats a great deal more carbohydrate than she needs to correct blood glucose levels, and/or attains excellent control of her blood glucose levels, she may, for example be a size 10–12. Teenage girls are very perceptive about diabetes and insulin. Significantly many teenage girls with type 1 diabetes recognise that, if they take insufficient insulin and run their blood glucose levels high, such as between 20 and 30 mmol/L, their bodies will break down fat and protein for energy so that over time they may lose too much weight and achieve a dress size of 2–4. Significant weight loss is an unfortunate goal of many teenage girls regardless of whether they have diabetes or not, but diabetes gives them a way to achieve it.

Uncontrolled diabetes can also result in a delayed onset of puberty and skeletal maturation (Silverstein *et al.* 2005). Studies have demonstrated higher rates of both anorexia and bulimia in young girls with type 1 diabetes (Jones *et al.* 2000). It is very important that health professionals are aware of the language they use when educating and advising young people with diabetes. References to weight can have devastating results. During the middle to late teenage years, the psychologist may be the most integral health professional on the diabetes team.

References

Abdul-Rasoul M, Habib H, Al-Khouly M (2006) The 'honeymoon phase' in children with type 1 diabetes mellitus: frequency, duration and influential factors. *Pediatric Diabetes* 7: 101–107.

American Association of Clinical Endocrinologists (2003) Position Statement: Inpatient Diabetes and Metabolic Control (www.aace.com/newsroom/press/2006/index.php/r=20060201)

American Diabetes Association (2004) Nutrition principles and recommendations in diabetes. *Diabetes Care* 27(1): S26–S46.

Annon J (1976) *Behavioural Treatment of Sexual Problems: Brief Therapy*. Harper and Row, New York.

Austroads (2006) Assessing fitness to drive: Austroads Guidelines for Health Professionals and Their Legal Obligations (2nd edn). APG56. Austroads, Sydney.

Bernstein L (2002) Post Menopausal Breast Cancer: Obesity and the Leptin Receptor. California Breast Cancer Research Program (www.cbcrp.org.research/PageGrant.asp/grant_id=1563).

Bethel MA, Sloan FA, Belsky D *et al.* (2007) Longitudinal incidence and prevalence of adverse outcomes of diabetes mellitus in elderly patients. *Archives of Internal Medicine* 167: 921–927.

Bosch J, Yusuf S, Gerstein HC *et al.* (DREAM Trial Investigators) (2006) Effect of ramipril on the incidence of diabetes. *New England Journal of Medicine* 355(15): 1551–1562.

Burchardt M, Burchardt T, Anastasiadis AG *et al.* (2002) Sexual dysfunction is common and overlooked in female patients with hypertension. *Journal of Sex and Marital Therapy* 28(1): 17–26.

Canadian Diabetes Association Clinical Practice Guidelines Expert Committee (2003) Clinical practice guidelines for the prevention and management of diabetes in Canada. *Canadian Journal of Diabetes* Suppl 2 (*www.diabetes.ca/cpg2003*).

Carnethon MR (2007) Depressive symptoms may be linked to risk for incident diabetes in older adults. *Medscape Medical News* (*www.medscape.com/viewarticle/555734*).

Chiasson JL, Josse RG, Gomis R *et al.* (STOP-NIDDM Trial Research Group) (2002) Acarbose treatment and the risk of cardiovascular disease and hypertension in patients with impaired glucose tolerance: the STOP–NIDDM trial. *Lancet* 359: 2072–2077.

Chisholm V, Atkinson L, Donaldson C *et al.* (2007) Predictors of treatment adherence in young children with type 1 diabetes. *Journal of Advanced Nursing* 57(5): 482–493.

Chong J, Craid M, Cameron F *et al.* (2007) Marked increase in type 1 diabetes mellitus incidence in children aged 0–14 yr in Victoria, Australia, from 1999 to 2002. *Pediatric Diabetes* 8(2): 67–73.

Colagiuri S, Cull C, Holman R (UKPDS Group) (2002) Are lower fasting plasma glucose levels at diagnosis associated with improved outcomes? UK Prospective Study 61. *Diabetes Care* 25(8): 1418–1424.

Craig M, Hattersley A, Donaghue K (2006) ISPAD clinical practice consensus guidelines 2006–2007: definition, epidemiology and classification. *Pediatric Diabetes* 7: 343–351.

Davis S, Renda M (2006) Psychological insulin resistance: overcoming barriers to starting insulin. *The Diabetes Educator* 32(4): 146s–152s.

Diabetes and Nutrition Study Group (DNSG) of the EASD (2004) Evidence-based nutritional approaches to the treatment and prevention of diabetes mellitus. *Nutrition Metabolism and Cardiovascular Diseases* 15: 373–394.

Diabetes Australia and the Royal Australian College of General Practitioners (RACGP) (2006) *Diabetes Management in General Practice 2005–2006*. RACGP, South Melbourne.

Dunning P (1993) Sexuality and women with diabetes. *International Patient Education and Counselling* 21: 5–14.

Dunstan D, Zimmet P, Welborn T (AusDiab Steering Committee) (2000) *Diabetes, Obesity and Associated Disorders in Australia 2000. The Accelerating Epidemic*. Australian Diabetes, Obesity and Lifestyle report. International Diabetes Institute, Melbourne.

Enzlin P, Mathieu C, Van den Bruel A *et al.* (2002) Sexual dysfunction in women with type 1 diabetes: a controlled study. *Diabetes Care* 25(4): 672–677.

Expert Committee on the Diagnosis and Classification of Diabetes Mellitus (1997) *Diabetes Care* 20: 1183–1197.

Hood K, Huestis S, Maher A *et al.* (2006) Children with type 1 diabetes often experience depressive symptoms. *Diabetes Care* 29: 1389–1391.

International Diabetes Federation (IDF) (2006) Incidence of diabetes. *Diabetes Atlas* 2006: 2 (*www.eatlas.idf.org/Incidence/*).

International Society for Pediatric and Adolescent Diabetes (ISPAD) (2000) Consensus Guidelines 2000: ISPAD Consensus Guidelines for the Management of Type 1 Diabetes Mellitus in Children and Adolescents. ISPAD, Berlin.

Jones J, Lawson M, Daneman D *et al.* (2000) Eating disorders in adolescent females with and without type 1 diabetes: cross sectional study. *British Medical Journal* 320: 1563–1566.

Khoo C, Mahesh P (2005) *Diabetes and the menopause.* Royal Society of Medicine Press 11(1): 6–11.

Knowler WC, Barrett-Connor E, Fowler SE *et al.* (Diabetes Prevention Program Research Group) (2002) Reduction in the incidence of type 2 diabetes with lifestyle intervention and metformin. *New England Journal of Medicine* 346: 393–403.

Maynard JD, Rohrscheib M, Way JF *et al.* (2007) Noninvasive type 2 diabetes screening: superior sensitivity to fasting plasma glucose and A1C. *Diabetes Care* 30(5): 1120–1124.

National Health and Medical Research Council (NHMRC) (2005) Evidence-based Guidelines for the Management of Type 2 Diabetes. NHMRC, Canberra (www.nhmrc.gov.au/publications/synopses/di7todi13syn.htm).

Naunheim R, Jang TJ, Banet G *et al.* (2006) Point-of-care test identifies diabetic ketoacidosis at triage. *Academic Emergency Medicine* 13: 683–685.

Nissen S, Wolski K (2007) Effect of rosiglitazone on risk of myocardial infarction and death from cardiovascular causes. *New England Journal of Medicine* 356(24): 2457–2471.

Ohl L (2007) Essentials of female sexual dysfunction from a sex therapy perspective. *Urology Nurse* 27(1): 57–63.

Pan XR, Li GW, Hu YH *et al.* (1997) Effects of diet and exercise in preventing NIDDM in people with impaired glucose tolerance. The Da Qiing IGT and Diabetes Study. *Diabetes Care* 20: 537–544.

Queensland Health (2002) Best Practice Guidelines for the Management of Type 1 Diabetes in Children and Adolescents. Queensland Health, Brisbane.

Salonia A, Briganti A, Montorsi P (2002) Sexual dysfunction in women with coronary artery disease. *International Journal of Impotence Research* 14(4): S80.

Schneider H (2006) Haemoglobin A1c measurement – pointers and pitfalls. *Diabetes Management Journal* 17: 26.

Schulze MB, Schulz M, Heidemann C *et al.* (2007) Fiber and magnesium intake protects against developing type 2 diabetes. *Archives of Internal Medicine* 167(9): 956–965.

Silink M (ed) (1996) APEG Handbook on Childhood and Adolescent Diabetes. APEG, Parramatta.

Silverstein J, Klingensmith G, Copeland K *et al.* (2005) Care of children and adolescents with type 1 diabetes: a statement of the American Diabetes Association. *Diabetes Care* 28(1): 186–212.

Tenolouris N (2006) Overview of diabetes. Chapter 1 in Katsilambros N, Diakoumopoulou E, Ioannidis I *et al.* (eds) *Diabetes in Clinical Practice.* John Wiley and Sons, Chichester, pp 1–21.

Tuomilehto J, Lindström J Eriksson J *et al.* (Finnish Diabetes Prevention Study Group) (2001) Prevention of type 2 diabetes by changes in lifestyle among subjects with impaired glucose tolerance. *New England Journal of Medicine* 344: 1343–1350.

United Kingdom Prospective Diabetes Study (UKPDS) 38 (1998) Tight blood pressure control and risk of macrovascular and microvascular complications in type 2 diabetes. *British Medical Journal* 317: 703–713.

World Health Organization (1999) *Diagnosis and Classification of Diabetes Mellitus.* WHO, Geneva.

Recommended reading

Australian Government Department of Health and Aging (2006) Australian Alcohol Guidelines (www.alcohol.gov.au/internet/alcohol/publishing.nsf/Content/guidelines).

Australian Medicines Handbook (2006) Rundle Mall, Adelaide.

Dunning T (2003) *Care of People with Diabetes. A Manual of Nursing Practice.* Blackwell Publishing, Oxford.

Ganz M (ed) (2005) *Prevention of Type 2 Diabetes.* John Wiley and Sons, Chichester.

Chapter 3

Health assessment, management targets, and deciding on a management plan

---

Key points

- Individualised holistic assessment is essential to planning appropriate care for people with diabetes.
- Mental, spiritual, and general health status should be monitored as assiduously as diabetes status.
- The individual must be involved in planning and monitoring his or her care.
- Collaborative, structured multidisciplinary team care is essential to achieving optimal outcomes and continuity of care.

Introduction

Major advances in understanding and managing diabetes continue to influence the way we manage and educate people with diabetes. Some major research milestones in the 20th century include the discovery of insulin in 1922, the development of the sulphonylureas in the 1950s, blood glucose self-monitoring products in 1978, and the advent of the HbA_{1c} assay. In the 21st century, blood glucose monitoring techniques and various assay methods are becoming more accurate, new oral hypoglycaemic agents, insulin analogues, lipid-lowering, and antihypertensive agents are being developed, and there is an ever-increasing amount of information about the pathophysiology, complications, and biochemistry that influence management and treatment targets.

In addition, psychological and education research demonstrates the critical importance of patient-centred care (see Chapter 8).

Management should be individualised, based on a careful assessment that includes the physical, psychological, cognitive, spiritual, knowledge, attitudes, beliefs, experience, and social and environmental factors that could affect an individual's self-care. Importantly, these factors need to be reassessed on a regular basis as diligently as screening for complications because they can change over time. In fact, such assessment should be part of the routine complication screening process. A good start towards incorporating these aspects into routine complication screening occurred in Australia when ANDIAB (Australian National Diabetes Information Audit and Benchmarking) 2 was introduced in 2006.

ANDIAB 1 is a long-term complication screening process and is part of a national complication screening programme. ANDIAB 2 addresses regular, structured diabetes education assessment. Such assessment is a proactive, preventive process that could help to predict future care requirements rather than just identifying complication rates and health professional compliance with guidelines. Significantly, spending time to develop a trusting relationship with the individual is essential, and is linked to better health outcomes.

The aims of diabetes management

The aims of management are to develop a management plan in collaboration with the multidisciplinary team, and, most importantly, support the individual to:

- achieve and maintain an acceptable weight;
- maintain physical activity and other activities of daily living (ADL) that are commensurate with the individual's desires, capabilities, and lifestyle;
- achieve an acceptable blood pressure. In people aged > 80 years, higher blood pressure is associated with longer 5-year survival rates than those with lower blood pressure in non-diabetics (Oates *et al.* 2007). The implications for people with diabetes are unclear. Some experts suggest the risk of vascular disease is significant at higher levels, especially in people with diabetes. The risk of postural hypotension contributing to falls in older people needs to be considered;
- normalise the blood glucose and lipid profiles. Suggested methods to reduce the discomfort of blood glucose monitoring are shown in Box 3.1;

- prevent short- and long-term complications by undertaking regular screening programmes and actively involving the individual in his/her care;
- limit the incidence and duration of the effects of intercurrent illness and the associated impact on metabolic control; and
- maintain psychological and spiritual well-being and quality of life (QoL).

Many validated tools exist to determine these issues and enable people to be compared with each other, especially in research projects. Patient-generated QoL, although they are not formally validated and may not enable people to be compared, can be scaled and assessed periodically to compare the person's QoL at different stages and may more closely represent the individual's specific QoL issues. That is they are valid for the particular individual (Jenkinson and McGee 1998). The current recommended management targets to achieve these aims are shown in Table 3.1, and Figure 3.1 is an example diabetes educator assessment sheet.

Box 3.1 Some suggestions that could help people with diabetes reduce the discomfort of home blood glucose monitoring

Most modern strips require a very small amount of blood to achieve an accurate result.

- Choose a lancet device that suits your needs. There are a number of different styles. The depth the lancet penetrates can be adjusted on some devices. Your diabetes educator can help you make an appropriate choice.
- The least painful spot is the sides of the fingertip and often it is the best spot to obtain an adequate drop of blood.
- Make sure the fingers are clean and dry before testing to reduce the possibility of contaminating the result with food and other substances. In addition, it is easier to obtain a drop of blood if the finger is warm.
- Alternate the fingers so you are not pricking the same finger or spot each time you test.
- Choose the most appropriate setting on the lancet to obtain a drop of blood. People who have a lot of callus from manual work usually require a deeper setting than those who do not.
- The lancet device should be pressed firmly against the side of the finger so the lancet penetrates easily. Keep the lancet pressed against the finger as you trigger the device.
- Use a new lancet each time you do a test and dispose of used lancets into an appropriate sharps container.

DATE:
AGE: TEL:
REFERRAL SOURCE AND DATE:
....

REASON FOR REFERRAL:

PATIENT GOAL/S:
COUNTRY OF BIRTH: PREFERRED LANGUAGE:
                                                     INTERPRETER REQUIRED?
LIVES WITH AND SOCIAL SUPPORT:
....
....

OCCUPATION:
INTERESTS:
FAMILY HISTORY: DM
GP:

MEDICAL MGMT.   ENDO ☐   DCAS ☐   GP ☐   OTHER ☐
NAME: _____

DATE OF DIAGNOSIS: TYPE: _____
CURRENT DIABETES TREATMENT:

                                                            SYRINGE   ☐
                                                            HUMAPEN   ☐
                                                            FLEXPEN   ☐
CURRENT SIGNS and SYMPTOMS   NOVOPEN 3   ☐
                                                            INNOLET   ☐
                                                            AUTOPEN 24   ☐
DKA/HYPO EVENTS and FREQUENCY: OTHER   ☐
                                                            NDSS   ☐

                                                            Sharps container   ☐

                          INJECTION SITES _____: Checked Y ☐ N ☐
NAME OF BG METER:
TESTING FREQUENCY and RESULTS:
OVERWEIGHT PRIOR TO DIAGNOSIS: Y ☐ N ☐
ACTIVITY LEVEL:

Current smoker: ☐   ALCOHOL: STRESS:
Ex smoker: ☐
Never smoked   ☐

SELF-COPING WITH DIABETES: (Not coping) **1** ————————————**10** (Coping)

Figure 3.1 Example diabetes assessment sheet.
Reproduced courtesy of Victoria Stevenson, Austin Health.

Figure 3.1 (*Continued*)

REPORTED GENERAL HEALTH:

OTHER MEDICATIONS (including over-the-counter medication)

LAST DIETITIAN REVIEW: _____

REGULARITY OF MEALS   B ☐   L ☐   D ☐
SNACKS: Y ☐   N ☐   SUPPER: Y ☐   N ☐

COMMENTS...

BGL today: _____   Time: _____

HbA$_{1c}$: ....   DATE: ....

LIPIDS: TC ____HDL-C _____TG _____   LDL-C_____   Date: _____

AER _____   eGFR _____ (Only reported if < 60)

WT _____   HT _____   HWR _____   BMI _____

WT GAIN: Y ☐ N ☐   LAST EYE CHECK _____
WT LOSS: Y ☐ N ☐   LAST POD CHECK _____
WT STABLE: Y ☐ N ☐

PREVIOUS ED. PROGRAMME/FEELINGS ABOUT COMMENCING
INSULIN/OTHER:
_____

ACTION TODAY:
_____
_____
_____
_____
_____
_____
_____

PLAN:
REFERRED TO: DIETITIAN ☐   PODIATRIST ☐   OTHER ☐
                 FURTHER DIAB EDUC. REQ.   YES ☐   NO ☐
AUSTIN HEALTH   ☐   DCAS ☐   NOT REQ. ☐

Diabetes Clinical Nurse Consultant
PAGER: ☐   ☐   ☐

Table 3.1 Diabetes management targets for people with diabetes. Specific management targets should be based on the individual's specific circumstances following an holistic assessment.

Management targets	Frequency of assessment
Control blood glucose $HbA_{1c} < 7\%$*	Self-capillary blood glucose monitoring ranges between 4 and 6–8 mmol/L for 90% of tests
	Measure HbA_{1c} twice a year if control is adequate
	Measure four times a year if control is inadequate or if the management regimen is adjusted frequently
Normalise blood lipids	Measure annually if within the target range
Cholesterol (LDL) < 2.5 mmol/L	Measure every 3–6 months if outside the range and familial hyperlipidaemia
Triglycerides < 2.0 mmol/L	
HDL > 1.0 mmol/L	
Control blood pressure – < 140/90 mmHg, 130/70 if renal disease is present	Measure every 3 months in people with hypertension†
	Measure every 6 months in normotensive people
Preserve renal function	Measure microalbumin annually or 3- to 6-monthly if microalbuminuria is detected
	Serum creatinine annually
Preserve vision	Eye examination at diagnosis in type 2 diabetes to determine presence of retinopathy. If no retinopathy, screen in 2 years
	If retinopathy is present, screen yearly. More frequent examinations may be needed
	Screen for macular degeneration in older people
	Assess need for and adequacy of glasses prescription (visual acuity)
Prevent foot pathology	Determine risk factors for foot ulceration
	Self foot checks regularly
	Assess both feet annually if no risk factors of pathology present
	Assess at least 3- to 6-monthly if at risk (see Chapter 7)
Monitor mental and physical function especially in older people	A range of measures can be used, such as: – MiniMental State Examination (MMSE) – Brief Case-Find For Depression (BCD) – Beck Depression Inventory (BDI) – Hospital Anxiety and Depression Scale (HADS)
Maintain meaning and quality of life (QoL)	QoL assessment tools such as SF-36 and ADDQoL, but consider using and monitoring patient-generated QoL

* Guidelines vary slightly in their recommendations: some recommend $HbA_{1c} < 6\%$, others < 6.5%.
† Some experts recommend measuring blood pressure at every visit. It is best to measure after the person relaxes during a consultation to reduce the effects of 'white coat hyperglycaemia'. Likewise the arm should be correctly positioned.

Smoking cessation

Stopping smoking is often a very difficult but essential aspect of diabetes management. Smoking is associated with a range of cardiovascular diseases, cancer, low bone density and premature death. In addition, passive smoking is associated with a number of diseases including exacerbation of respiratory diseases, coronary heart disease and death in non-smokers (Surgeon General's Report 2006). Nicotine addiction is a chronic relapsing disease and the average smoker quits several times (Wise *et al.* 2007). Long-term counselling and support are required to help people quit. A range of pharmacologic therapies is available if other strategies are ineffective. These include various nicotine preparations (gum, patches, lozenges, nasal spray), bupropion and varenicline.

Monitoring the effectiveness of the management plan

Regular blood glucose self-monitoring (BGSM) is one way to involve the individual in his or her care, determine the effectiveness of the management regimen, and make adjustments if necessary. BGSM results must be considered in conjunction with biochemical parameters such as HbA_{1c}, lipids, food intake, and activity levels because there is ample evidence that BGSM results are inaccurate (Natrass 2002). Despite these limitations, BGSM is an important way of involving the individual in his/her care. The fact that they record incorrect results does not mean they do not recognise the significance of the results.

Blood glucose monitoring is particularly important in the following circumstances:

- frequent hypoglycaemia including nocturnal hypoglycaemia;
- during prolonged stress or illness where insulin may be needed
  - in people with type 2 diabetes on oral glucose-lowering agents (OHA) (rescue therapy)
  - during pregnancy
  - in women with gestational diabetes
  - during hospitalisation
- when managing intercurrent illnesses at home;
- when a new treatment regimen is commenced, for example insulin is added to the OHA regimen;
- when the person has complications such as renal failure, autonomic neuropathy, cardiovascular disease or cerebrovascular insufficiency.

Hypoglycaemia can be masked and the symptoms may not be recognised in these circumstances; and

- diabetes in pregnancy and gestational diabetes.

When interpreting blood glucose levels, it is important to consider the total picture, which includes factors such as:

- the time the test was performed;
- BGSM testing accuracy;
- the type of diet the person consumes;
- exercise;
- medication self-management practices;
- presence of intercurrent illness such as influenza and urinary tract infection;
- the presence of renal, liver and pancreatic disease;
- unrelieved pain or stress;
- use of other medicines such as glucocorticoids and complementary and non-prescription medications, especially those that contain glucose, ephedrine, pseudoephedrine, or alcohol, for example cold remedies; and
- alcohol consumption.

BGSM frequency depends on individual circumstances and varies from daily to four to six times per day. More frequent testing such as two-hourly is recommended during illness and blood ketone levels should also be monitored during illness especially in the presence of hyperglycaemia and in type 1 diabetes (see Chapter 6). Many people report that BGSM is painful: some ways to reduce the discomfort are shown in Box 3.1.

There is also some debate about the relative value of fasting and postprandial BGSM testing and the timing of postprandial testing – that is, testing during the immediate post-absorptive state or after 2–3 hours. The postprandial state lasts up to 5 hours, so undertaking three postprandial tests per day reflects 70% of the prevailing blood glucose level (Del Prato 2002). However, a number of factors influence postprandial glucose levels, including:

- loss of first phase insulin secretion, a common feature of type 2 diabetes (see Chapter 2);
- the degree of insulin resistance in muscle and adipose tissue, which is associated with obesity and prolonged stress;
- gastric emptying time, which is influenced by a number of factors including diet and the presence of autonomic neuropathy;
- inadequate suppression of gluconeogenesis, for example during prolonged physical or psychological stress; and

- the presence of free fatty acids, which may occur during illness and hyperglycaemia (Del Prato and Tiengo 2001).

Postprandial glucose is the major contributor to HbA_{1c} levels in the normal range. The contribution of fasting glucose increases as the fasting blood glucose level increases. Therefore, fasting and postprandial BGSM tests provide different and equally important information. Postprandial glucose may predict the likelihood of complications developing and is an independent predictor of cardiovascular mortality in type 2 diabetes, even increases as low as 1% (Hanefeld *et al.* 1996).

Holistic health assessment

The individual's diabetes-specific status should be assessed on a regular basis as follows:

- regular weight checks (and/or BMI and waist circumference) to estimate loss or gain and compare with the weight management goal. South Asian, North American Aboriginal and Chinese ethnicity appear to be associated with abnormal glucose and lipid levels and blood pressure at a lower BMI. Ethnic differences should be considered when assessing weight;
- lying and standing blood pressure to detect any postural drop, which could indicate autonomic neuropathy. In older people postural hypotension contributes to falls risk;
- retinal screening and visual acuity. Visual acuity needs to be interpreted according to blood glucose level and age. High and low blood glucose levels can cause changes in the lens that make many routine practices such as reading difficult but are not sight threatening. Macular degeneration is a common cause of visual loss in older people;
- cardiovascular assessment including the feet (see Chapter 7);
- peripheral neuropathy (see Chapter 7);
- kidney function such as microalbuminuria, creatinine clearance, and the albumin/creatinine ratio, which need to be interpreted according to the individual's age and gender;
- insulin injection sites;
- regular assessment of diabetes knowledge about:
  - diet;
  - self-care techniques; and
  - the individual's (and his or her carer's) general health care and diabetes-specific knowledge and beliefs and attitudes;
- quality of life, depression, and cognitive ability especially in older people;

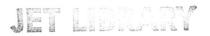

- regular structured medication review including over-the-counter and complementary therapy (CAM) use. Medicines should be reviewed when a new medicine is introduced. A home medicines review might be indicated (see Chapter 5).

In addition, the status of existing comorbidities and the development of new ones should be part of the assessment.

General health assessment includes:

- Papanicolaou smear
- mammography
- tests of prostate function
- immunisation status, especially in at-risk groups such as older people and children
- dental health.

A systematic recent review of the relevant literature indicates that general health assessment or 'medical check-up' is associated with improvements in delivering some recommended preventive services and less worry for patients (Boulware *et al.* 2007). Often, these aspects are not part of routine diabetes complication or risk assessment practices, which can lead to fragmented and uncoordinated care and/or inadequate screening and monitoring.

Laboratory assessments

Glycosylated haemoglobin (HbA$_{1c}$)

HbA$_{1c}$ is the most frequently used test of metabolic control, but it is not used to diagnose diabetes. It is a reliable indicator of the average blood glucose level over the preceding 3 months and forms when haemoglobin is exposed to circulating blood glucose. HbA$_{1c}$ corresponds with circulating blood glucose representing approximately 50% in the first month and 25% in the second and third months. A number of assay methods are used and it is most useful if the individual attends the same laboratory for each test.

In addition, the HbA$_{1c}$ level can be affected:

- reduced survival time of red blood cells, anaemia, and abnormal transferrins can result in lower HbA$_{1c}$;
- the presence of fetal haemoglobin or sickle cells can lead to lower levels;
- the presence of carbamylated haemoglobin, which occurs in uraemic syndromes, can lead to higher levels;

- hypoglycaemia, recent blood loss, and blood transfusions can also lead to lower levels.

HbA_{1c} is usually tested at least 3 months apart but can be done sooner to gauge the effect of a treatment modification. A change of 0.5% reflects a true change. HbA_{1c}can be performed on a fingerprick blood sample at the consultation, which enables the information to be used proactively during the consultation and timely adjustments to the management regimen to be made.

Serum lipids

Hyperglycaemia and elevated serum lipids are usually present together. In particular, cholesterol, low density lipoprotein, and triglycerides are high, and high density lipoprotein is low; a situation that predisposes the individual to cardiovascular events. Fasting blood samples are most useful and are generally preferred. Lipids consist of:

- cholesterol;
- triglycerides;
- lipoproteins, which consist of:
  - very low density lipoprotein (VLDL);
  - low density lipoprotein (LDL); and
  - high density lipoprotein (HDL).

Type 2 diabetes is typically associated with elevated cholesterol and triglycerides and low HDL, which is atherogenic and contributes to vascular risk.

C-peptide

Endogenous insulin consists of two chains. C-peptide determines the folding of the two insulin chains during insulin production and storage in the pancreas. It splits off in the final stages and can be measured to determine whether endogenous insulin production is still occurring and to distinguish between type 1 and type 2 diabetes, if the difference is not clear from the clinical presentation, for example lean older people.

Other tests

Other tests used to confirm type 1 diabetes are:

- islet cell antibodies (ICA), which are present before the clinical signs of diabetes appear; and
- GAD antibodies, which are present in 80% of people with type 1 diabetes (Cohen 1996). It is important to distinguish between type 1 and type 2 diabetes so that appropriate management strategies can be implemented (see Chapter 2).

Tests of kidney function

Creatinine clearance, serum creatinine, albumin/creatinine ratio, glomerular filtration rate, and blood urea nitrogen (BUN) are used to estimate renal function and nutritional status (protein), screen for renal function decline, and determine whether parenteral nutrition and dialysis are required. More recently, the estimated glomerular filtration rate (eGFR) is becoming more widely used. The eGFR takes into account age and gender and, although not perfect, it is a more accurate indicator of renal function than serum creatinine alone.

Twelve and 24-hour urine collections are used to calculate creatinine clearance rates and microalbumin excretion rates. Microalbumin is present in the early stages of renal damage, well before protein appears. Recently, machines that measure urinary albumin at the time of the consultation were introduced. They are an important indicator of early kidney disease and predict cardiovascular damage. Early diagnosis and treatment can delay the onset of nephropathy and the need for dialysis by 24 years, which in turn increases life expectancy and maintains quality of life (Borch-Johnsen *et al.* 1993; see Chapter 7).

Multidisciplinary team care and shared care

Modern diabetes management requires a collaborative multidisciplinary team approach combined with adequate self-care. The person with diabetes is a central and essential team member. Team care means health professional disciplines complement each other, may have overlapping roles, and are interdependent in the way they support the person with diabetes. Team or shared care also refers to continuity of care between various service providers such as acute and community care and among team members. It helps achieve seamless coordinated care, avoid duplicated services, improve communication, and standardise care.

CASE DISCUSSION

> **Mrs PC**
>
> ***Mrs PC was referred to a tertiary diabetes clinic by a practice nurse (nurse working in a general practice)***
> Can you help me sort out this confusing issue both for the GPs and for myself? I have encouraged the GPs that I work for to allow the older patients to run their BGLs higher rather than lower. Consequently, I saw a 75-year-old lean type 2 woman, who had limited exercise ability, was maintaining a healthy diet, not on OHAs, and had a HbA_{1c} of 7.7%. She uses a walking frame and I thought this was OK. My confusion arises with the older people when their BGs are between 5 and 7 mmol/L and the HbA_{1c} is above 7% and the GP says we need to improve the HbA_{1c}, especially as many older patients have other illnesses, and impairment in speech, mobility, or understanding. Many of them eat like church mice and the GPs still want to push for unrealistic goals.
>   Help please.

Diabetes educator

The most important 'take-home' message about HbA_{1c} is that it is only one part of the overall picture and does not tell us everything (see Chapter 2). We need to avoid making clinical decisions about diabetes targets on chronological age rather than according to the level of functioning, the wishes of the patient, and the degree of support they have. It may be appropriate to use a short-acting sulphonylurea such as glicazide or the long-acting glicazide modified release (MR) that only acts when the blood glucose levels rise in healthy older people with few comorbidities and a positive approach to healthy ageing.

Lean older people are unlikely to have significant insulin resistance, and, therefore, will probably not benefit from metformin or a thiazolidinedione. Metformin is generally contraindicated in people over the age of 80 years due to a higher risk of lactic acidosis, which has up to a 50% mortality rate. Metformin can reduce appetite in older people who often have nutritional deficiencies and may need to eat more. Acarbose does not usually cause hypoglycaemia but it only lowers HbA_{1c} by 0.5% and is often not tolerated because it causes flatulence.

We need to consider what we hope to achieve by reducing Mrs PC's HbA_{1c} to 7%. Controlling blood pressure and lipids is also necessary to prevent long-term diabetes complications. Lower blood glucose levels in frail, at-risk older people may significantly reduce quality of life and safety by increasing the risk of falls and hypoglycaemia, which affects cognitive functioning and independence. That is not to say that we allow blood glucose levels to remain > 15 mmol/L all the time because that carries a risk of dehydration, polyuria, lethargy, intercurrent infections, falls, and hyperosmolar states. Mrs PC uses a walking frame, which puts her in the high-risk falls category.

Although the treatment of type 2 diabetes is diet, exercise, and medication, in older people these treatments need to be considered by asking the following questions:

(1) Is it safe?
(2) Does it make sense?
(3) Will it enhance the person's quality of life?

GPs try to do the right thing for their patients. They are under tremendous pressure to ensure that all their patients reach the desired management targets including HbA_{1c} < 7%. Age-related factors are rarely considered when glycaemic goals are discussed. For example, endocrinologists tolerate much higher HbA_{1c} levels in infants and young children with type 1 diabetes than older children, due to the risk of unpredictable hypoglycaemia. The same principle can be applied to frailer older people. People with diabetes are more than their HbA_{1c} level. Good communication and education between GPs, practice nurses, and diabetes specialists enables more realistic goals to be negotiated. These goals can be identified and articulated using General Practitioner Management Plans (Enhanced Primary Care Items, Australia) (Australian Diabetes Educators Association *et al.* 2007).

Dietitian

I would discuss what the GP sees as the advantages of improving glycaemic control in this woman and ask him or her to consider the disadvantages, most of which were outlined by the Diabetes Educator. I would like more information about how long Mrs PC has had diabetes and her glycaemic history. I also need to know her complication status and whether any complications she has are being treated, whether they affect her quality of life, and whether improving her glycaemic control would prevent them deteriorating.

I wonder whether she has episodes of hypoglycaemia. Tightening her control might exacerbate or precipitate hypoglycaemia. It is also important to determine whether her poor control is causing symptoms such as thirst, polyuria, infections, tiredness and fatigue. She may need education about how to manage her diabetes and we should identify what her wishes are. I would advise Mrs PC to attend structured diabetes self-management education if she is willing to, and include her carers in the education.

I would advise the GP to discuss the issues with her family by informing them of the risks and benefits of tight control.

CASE DISCUSSION

> ***Question from a nurse working in an aged care facility***
> I am an RN (registered nurse) working in aged care. One resident is ordered Humalog but I only have NovoRapid in stock.
>   Can I use these insulins interchangeably?

Diabetes educator

Both these insulins are rapid-acting insulin analogues used to treat type 1 and type 2 diabetes. They have a similar action profile, but research suggests there may be differences between them. Humalog (lispro) is absorbed and eliminated more rapidly than NovoRapid, but the blood glucose-lowering effect is similar (Hedman *et al.* 2001). The clinical significance of this finding is unclear. Another study in 'healthy volunteers' showed that NovoRapid had a more rapid onset of action and a higher peak (von Mach *et al.* 2002). The action profile is likely to vary among individuals and within individuals depending on factors at any given time (e.g. illness, injection site). Glulisine (Apidra) is available in some countries and could be more rapidly absorbed than Humalog or NovoRapid.

The insulins may be interchangeable, but doing so is not recommended. If you do substitute NovoRapid for Humalog, monitor the blood glucose after the change and do not alternate between the two insulins.

CASE DISCUSSION

> **Mr WWB**
>
> ***Mr WWB was referred to the diabetes educator by a nurse working on a medical ward***
> We have a man here on the medical ward with COAD (chronic obstructive airways disease). He is in a bad way and was commenced on steroids to control the COAD. Now his blood glucose has gone very high.
>   Can you please give him some education about diabetes and suggest how we treat him. We are giving him stat doses of Actrapid when his glucose is over 10, usually after lunch.

Diabetes educator

There are three types of steroids:

- mineralocorticoid;
- glucocorticoid; and
- androgens/oestrogens.

Mr WWB was most likely prescribed a glucocorticoid, which reduces insulin release from the pancreatic beta cells at high doses, increases insulin resistance in the liver and muscle, stimulates gluconeogenesis, and increases hepatic glucose output, all of which lead to hyperglycaemia. Obesity and family history of diabetes increase the risk of developing diabetes when steroids are needed. Glucocorticoids might also affect intracellular glucose transport. The diabetogenic effects may be temporary if a specific course of steroids is needed but recur if the dose is increased or steroids are used intermittently. The risk of developing glucose intolerance or diabetes with glucocorticoid use increases if there is a family history of diabetes and obesity and other diabetes risk factors are present.

The specific steroid prescribed, the duration of the course, frequency of the dose, and treatment schedule were not provided and need to be considered when determining whether glucose-lowering medicines are indicated. However, glucose intolerance can occur within 48 hours of commencing steroids. Alternate day, interrupted dose regimes, short courses, and IV administration have less impact on blood glucose than long-term high-dose regimens. Hypertension, suppressed immune function, osteoporosis, and mood changes are other significant side effects that need to be considered and managed.

Mr WWB's blood glucose pattern, where the blood glucose increases over the course of the day, is not unusual. Blood glucose monitoring should be continued, probably before each meal and before bed until the blood glucose pattern stabilises. If the steroid dose is short-term (7–14 days), twice-a-day insulin or a long-acting insulin analogue might be needed. If long-term steroids are indicated, oral glucose-lowering agents might be effective if there are no contraindications to their use. Top doses of insulin are not recommended. They are reactive and only partially correct the blood glucose.

If Mr WWB is discharged on steroids he will need careful education about how to manage his steroids, including managing his glucose-lowering medicines if the steroid dose is increased or reduced. He will need to learn blood glucose testing, safe sharps disposal, how and where to obtain his diabetic supplies, and should carry a card indicating he has diabetes and that he is on steroid medicines. He should be advised to have relevant immunisations to prevent intercurrent infections such as influenza, and a complication assessment, and may benefit from a dietetic review.

Atypical antipsychotic medicines are also associated with hyperglycaemia and diabetes (Guo *et al.* 2006).

CASE DISCUSSION

> **Mr XYZ**
>
> **Mr XYZ was referred by his GP**
> I saw Mr XYZ today for a routine checkup. He is basically well but is complaining of putting on a lot of weight since you started him on insulin 6 months ago. He said about 7 kg. He is trying with his diet and exercise and his glucose control is reasonable.
>   Can you please advise him what to do?

Diabetes educator

The UK Prospective Diabetes Study (UKPDS) showed that every 1% reduction in HbA_{1c} reduced the risk of microvascular complications by 30% but increased the risk of hypoglycaemia by 25% and was associated with an average weight gain of approximately 2 kg/1% reduction in HbA_{1c} (UKPDS 1998). Putting on weight is one of the reasons many people with type 2 diabetes do not want to start insulin. Some weight gain occurs initially when the blood glucose control improves and the glucose that was previously excreted in the urine begins entering the cells. This could account for the weight increase Mr XYZ describes.

Sulphonylureas and thiazolidinediones also increase weight, and consideration could be given to stopping these medicines if he is still taking them. Another possibility that needs to be considered is that he might be having hypoglycaemia associated with his exercise and eating more food to treat it, which in turn contributes to weight gain. If that is the case, his insulin regime may need to be adjusted and education about exercising safely provided.

I would check whether he is also taking other medicines that contribute to weight gain such as some atypical antipsychotic medicines, and check his thyroid status.

I would refer him to a dietitian for dietary advice and suggest exercise strategies such as wearing a pedometer, with the aim of gradually increasing his exercise level, and educate him about caring for his feet during exercise.

CASE DISCUSSION

> **Mr TME**
>
> ***Telephone question from a nurse on a medical ward***
> Just a quick question about Mr TME. His blood glucose is regularly about 4 mmol/L before breakfast on the ward.
>   Should I withhold his insulin? My colleagues said we should, and treat him for a hypo.

Diabetes educator

A blood glucose level of 4 mmol/L before breakfast indicates that the current insulin regimen and doses are effective and his blood glucose is in the pre-meal target range. The evening or pre-bed insulin is largely responsible for the pre-breakfast level. Mr TME should be given his insulin, followed immediately by his breakfast if he is prescribed a rapid-acting analogue. Withholding his insulin is likely to result in hyperglycaemia before lunch. If he is older and at risk of falling it might be necessary to adjust the dose of his evening insulin or ensure he has supper to achieve a pre-breakfast blood glucose of approximately 6 mmol/L.

Dietitian

A blood glucose reading of 4 mmol/L is at the lower end of the normal range. It should be acceptable to give Mr TME his insulin as long as it is immediately followed by breakfast. However, if the level is frequently < 4 mmol/L, the evening dose should be reduced.

References

Australian Diabetes Educators Association, Dietitians Association of Australia, Australian Association for Exercise and Sports Science (2007) *Type 2 Diabetes Medicare Group Services Information Pack*. Canberra.

Borch-Johnsen K, Wenzel H, Vibert G *et al.* (1993) Is screening and intervention for microalbuminuria worthwhile in patients with IDDM? *British Medical Journal* 306: 1722–1725.

Boulware LE, Marinopoulos S, Phillips KA *et al.* (2007) Systematic review. The value of the periodic health examination. *Annals of Internal Medicine* 146: 289–300.

Cohen M (1996) *Diabetes: A Handbook of Management.* International Diabetes Institute, Melbourne.

Del Prato S (2002) In search of normoglycaemia in diabetes: controlling postprandial glucose. *International Journal of Obesity* 26: s 9–17.

Del Prato S, Tiengo A (2001) The importance of first-phase insulin secretion: implications for the therapy of type 2 diabetes. *Diabetes Metabolism Research Review* 17: 164–174.

Guo JJ, Keck PE Jr, Corey-Lisle PK *et al.* (2006) Risk of diabetes mellitus associated with atypical antipsychotic use among patients with bipolar disorder: a retrospective, population-based case-control study. *Journal of Clinical Psychiatry* 67: 1055.

Hanefeld M, Fischer S, Julius U *et al.* (1996) The DIS-Group: risk factors for myocardial infarction and death in newly diagnosed NIDDM: the diabetes intervention study, 11-year follow-up. *Diabetologia* 29: 2072–2077.

Hedman C, Lindstrom T, Arnqvist H (2001) Direct comparison of insulin aspart and insulin lispro in patients with type 1 diabetes. *Diabetes Care* 24: 1120–1121.

Jenkinson C, McGee H (1998) *Health Status Measurement: A Brief But Critical Introduction.* Radcliffe Medical Press, Oxford, pp 61–63.

Natrass M (2002) Improving results from home blood-glucose monitoring: accuracy and reliability require greater patient education as well as improved technology. *Clinical Chemistry* 48: 979–980.

Oates D, Berlowitz D, Glickman M *et al.* (2007) Blood pressure survival in the oldest old. *Journal of the American Geriatrics Society* 55(3): 383–388.

Surgeon General's Report (2006) *The Health Consequences of Involuntary Exposure to Tobacco Smoke: A Report of the Surgeon General – Executive Summary.* US Department of Health and Human Services, Centre for Disease Control and Prevention, Office of Smoking and Health.

UK Prospective Diabetes Study Group (1998) Intensive blood glucose control with sulphonylureas or insulin compared with conventional treatment and risk of complications in patients with type 2 diabetes. UKPDS 33. *Lancet* 52: 837–853.

Von Mach M, Brinkmann C, Hansen T *et al.* (2002) Differences in pharmacokinetics and pharmacodynamics of insulin lispro and aspart in health volunteers. *Experimental Clinical Endocrinology and Diabetes* 110: 416–419.

Wise G, Sims T, Taylor R (2007) Smoking cessation – a practical guide for the physician. *Primary Care Reports* 13(4): 49–60.

Recommended reading

Abrahamson M (2004) Optimal glycaemic control in type 2 diabetes mellitus. Fasting postprandial context. *Archives of Internal Medicine* 164: 486–491.

Australian Medicines Handbook (2006) National Prescribing Service, Adelaide.

Bergenstal RM, Gavin JR (2005) The role of blood glucose self-monitoring in the care of people with diabetes: report of a global consensus conference. *American Journal of Medicine* 118(9a): 1S–6S.

British Diabetes Association (1999) *Guidelines for Practice for Residents with Diabetes in Care Homes.* Diabetes UK, London.

Diabetes Control and Complications Trial (DCCT) Research Group (1993) Effects of intensive insulin therapy on the development and progression of long-term complications of IDDM. *New England Journal of Medicine* 329: 977–986.

Dunning T (2003) *Care of People with Diabetes: A Manual of Nursing Practice.* Blackwell Publishing, Oxford.

Dunning T (2005) *Nursing Care of Older People with Diabetes.* Blackwell Publishing, Oxford.

National Heart Foundation (2001) *Lipid Management Guidelines.* National Heart Foundation, Melbourne.

UK Prospective Study Group (1998) Intensive blood glucose control with sulphonylureas or insulin compared with conventional treatment and risk of complications in patients with type 2 diabetes. UKPDS 33. *Lancet* 52: 837–853.

Chapter 4

Nutritional management and physical activity

Key points

- Good nutrition and appropriate physical activity are essential to good health and diabetes management.
- Nutrition and physical activity are still essential when oral glucose-lowering agents and/or insulin is required.
- Malnutrition is common despite obesity, especially in older people.
- People's food beliefs and the social and cultural aspects of food need to be considered.
- People who present with other comorbidities such as disordered eating, renal or gastrointestinal diseases require assessment by a dietitian.
- Changing people's eating behaviour is difficult – behavioural approaches, motivational interviewing, goal setting, and lifestyle counselling are essential to dietary change.

Introduction

Nutritional management and physical activity, the so-called lifestyle interventions, are essential to achieving optimal health and well-being, preventing type 2 diabetes (see Chapter 2), and achieving diabetes management targets regardless of the diabetes type. They remain essential even when medicines are needed. Prevention studies show that lifestyle interventions confer lasting benefits (Da Quing Study (Pan *et al.* 1997); Finnish Diabetes Prevention Study (Tuomilehto *et al.* 2001); US Diabetes Prevention Programme (Knowler *et al.* 2001)). These studies suggest that risk reduction was largely due to weight reduction, reducing fat intake, increasing fibre intake, and exercise. Obesity is linked to a range of diseases besides type 2 diabetes including coronary heart disease, gall bladder disease, cancer, and osteoarthritis.

The focus should be on eating a variety of nutritious foods every day to meet the individual's nutrient requirements, considering food preferences, religious, cultural, and social needs. The diet should aim to reduce cardiovascular risk and prevent obesity. Table 4.1 outlines the dietary recommendations from Europe, the USA, UK and Australia. Common recommendations include:

- Limit the intake of saturated fats/trans fatty acids to < 7% of total energy needs and cholesterol to < 200 mg/day.
- Consume adequate protein foods that contain essential amino acids to maintain normal growth and repair, hormone production, and renal function, 15–20% of total energy intake. High protein diets to achieve weight loss are not recommended.
- Include plenty of wholegrain cereals, bread and pasta (50–60% of total intake) especially foods with a low glycaemic index (GI). Carbohydrate balance is the key to metabolic control and very low carbohydrate diets are not recommended.
- Eat plenty of fruit and vegetables to reduce the risk of cardiovascular disease and degenerative diseases and supply essential vitamins and minerals such as chromium, calcium, zinc and antioxidants and flavonoids.
- Have adequate fluid intake, especially water, unless fluid restriction is indicated.
- Drink alcohol in moderation. Alcohol should be consumed with food to reduce the risk of hypoglycaemia when insulin or glucose-lowering oral agents are required. Moderate consumption of alcohol might have health benefits.
- Choose low salt foods and only add small amounts of salt to food (National Health and Medical Research Council 1999).
- Consider the medicine regimen and foods that could interact with medicines and nutrients whose absorption could be affected by medicines or affect the absorption or metabolism of medicines, and foods that are considered to be medicines (see Chapter 11).

Long-term hyperglycaemia can lead to nutritional deficiencies (Mooradian *et al.* 1994) and if the dietary intake cannot be improved, supplements may be required for:

- older people
- vegans
- pregnant women
- people who do not spend enough time outside or who cover up when outside.

However, despite the evidence that oxidative stress contributes to the development of diabetes complications, there is limited evidence

Table 4.1 Summary of nutritional guidelines. All recommend a carbohydrate intake between 50 and 70% of total energy intake. Sucrose does not necessarily need to be restricted. Up to 10% of the total daily energy derived from carbohydrate is acceptable. Monounsaturated fats (MUFA) are preferred to saturated and trans-unsaturated fatty acids, which should provide less than 10% of total energy. Polyunsaturated fats (PUFA) should not exceed 10%.

	Europe	USA	UK	Australia
Energy	If overweight: energy deficit of 500 kcal/day for a 10-kg weight loss	Standard weight reduction diets Added exercise and behaviour strategies are essential for long-term success	If overweight: energy deficit of 500 kcal/day, aiming to achieve 1- to 2-kg weight loss/month	If overweight: energy deficit of 500 kcal/day, aiming to achieve 1- to 2-kg weight loss/month
Carbohydrate	High in fibre, low GI recommended, as well as vegetables, fruits and cereals	Total carbohydrate content of meals/snacks more important than GI. Whole grain foods, fruit, vegetables and low fat milk	Actively promote low-GI foods	Actively promote low-GI foods and recommend carbohydrate comprises 50% of total energy intake
Protein	10–20% of total kcal or 0.8 kg/kg body weight if microalbuminuria is present	15–20% of total daily energy intake Requirements may be higher if metabolic control is poor		10–20% of total energy
Fat	Dietary cholesterol intake less than 300 mg/day Oily fish consumption recommended	Dietary cholesterol intake less than 300 mg/day Oily fish supplements to reduce triglyceride levels	Oily fish consumption recommended	< 30% of total energy intake, foods low in saturated fats and high in omega-3 or omega-6 polyunsaturated fats are recommended to reduce cholesterol, triglycerides and LDL
Alcohol	The equivalent of 1–2 glasses of wine/day is acceptable Drink with food if on sulphonylureas or insulin	No more than two alcohol drinks/day One drink represents 16 g alcohol and is equivalent to 12 oz beer, 5 oz wine, 15 oz spirits	Sensible drinking for the whole population: maximum 14 units/week for women and 21 units/week for men with 1–2 alcohol-free days/week	Minimal intake; < 4 standard drinks/day for men and < 2 standard drinks/day for women
Physical activity	Walk 4 hours/week to achieve a 2000 kcal/week deficit	30 minutes of moderate physical activity on most days	20–30 minutes of physical activity on most days	Aerobic exercise 3–4 times/week for 30 minutes/session 150 minutes of moderate physical activity – such as walking – per week (30 minutes over 5 or more days)

GI, glycaemic index; LDL, low density lipoprotein

that antioxidant supplementation is beneficial (American Diabetes Association 2006).

The nutrition plan should be revised regularly because requirements change: for example, as a child grows and develops, in older age, during pregnancy, when medications change, complications/comorbidities develop, and during intercurrent illness or surgery. It is important to check assumptions, for example there is an assumption that vegetarians eat high fibre/high carbohydrate diets. While that may be the case in their country of origin, once they migrate they frequently consume high quantities of energy-dense and saturated fat foods (Peterson and Govindji 1988).

An exercise or 'keep active' programme is also essential to good health and managing diabetes. Importantly, nutritional status is influenced by many factors including knowledge about food, shopping habits, methods of storing and preparing food, financial constraints, limited mobility and vision, and social factors such as living alone and living in residential care facilities. People may need information about coping with these issues as well as nutrition information relevant to their culture and lifestyle, attitudes, and food beliefs.

Obesity

Obesity is common in people with type 2 diabetes, and the prevalence of both obesity and type 2 diabetes is increasing, including in children. Obesity usually occurs as a result of eating excess amounts of energy-dense foods, lack of exercise, excess alcohol intake, some medicines and more rarely some endocrine diseases such as Cushing's disease. Obesity is now considered to be a disease in its own right (Marks 2000). Forty to sixty per cent of obesity may be inherited through an obesity gene expressed in adipose tissue; more likely there are hundreds of genes that influence body weight, so that both genes and the environment influence weight (Chagnon *et al.* 2000; Bouchard *et al.* 2004). Most obese people are deficient in leptin, a hormone that plays a key role in modulating appetite and the metabolic rate. Abdominal obesity significantly increases the risk of obesity-related diseases such as diabetes, dyslipidaemia, hypertension, vascular disease, fatty liver, and some cancers. Visceral fat confers the highest risk, followed by abdominal fat.

Measuring obesity can be difficult in clinical situations. A range of measures is used and they each have advantages and disadvantages. Crude weight compared to height/weight charts is a useful measure in most clinical situations. Body mass index (BMI) is regarded as a measure of central obesity, but it may not be as useful for individuals because it might 'discriminate against muscular men' (Egger 2007) but BMI > 30 usually indicates excess adipose tissue (Moyad 2007). Waist circumference might be preferable – < 100 cm for men and < 85 cm for women (Egger 2007). Waist circumference also varies between people from different ethnic groups, and factors such as standing position, time of the day the measurement is made and inspiration depth affect the measurement to an unknown degree (Moyad 2007). Changes in hydration status, and the presence of oedema and ascites can also affect waist–hip measurements. In addition, weight loss can be masked by oedema. Less commonly used measures include bioelectrical impedance, densitometry, dual energy X-ray absorptiometry (DEXA), and lean body mass.

Obesity is a significant global health problem associated with lifestyle factors such as calorie dense foods and inactivity compounding genetic predisposition. World Health Organization data suggest that 70% of the world's population is overweight (International Diabetes Federation 2006). The Australian Institute of Health and Welfare (AIHW) suggests that 56% of Australians are overweight (2006). A recent *Australian Doctor*/Pfizer survey indicates that the public believes obesity is a significant health problem (76% of *n* = 1300); but only 31% (35% women and 26% males) consider themselves to be overweight or obese (Howe 2007). Respondents indicated that eating less junk food, encouraging children to exercise and teaching them healthy eating habits are essential to reducing obesity. They indicated that health warnings about 'fattening food' were less important.

Addressing obesity is an essential aspect of managing diabetes, because type 2 diabetes and many other health problems coexist. However, it is important to consider the individual's specific nutritional needs rather than just providing them with a 'weight loss plan,' 'diabetic diet,' a 'standard meal plan' or information about 'healthy eating.' Considering nutrition rather than 'a diet' is more in keeping with holistic care. Obesity is a chronic condition and long-term holistic approach to management and a great deal of support are required to achieve weight loss. Motivational interviewing appears to be an effective strategy in women with type 2 diabetes, in addition to other strategies (West 2007).

Low-calorie diets and weight loss medicines

In some circumstances, very low calorie food substitutes such as Modifast might be considered, but their use needs to be balanced against the need for adequate nutrition and the ability to maintain such diets in the long term. Reviewing the need for medicines and diseases that contribute to weight gain is important. Using weight loss medicines may have a role to complement – but not replace – lifestyle measures. They should be used in the short term under supervision to reduce weight quickly or overcome 'the plateau' (Egger 2007). Currently available weight loss medicines are lipase inhibitors such as Xenical (orlistat) and serotonin reuptake inhibitors such as sibutramide and phentemine, which are not recommended in some guidelines because of the possibility of addiction. Another weight loss medicine, rimonabant, may be available in the near future. If Xenical (orlistat) is used, providing a low-fat diet is essential. Dietary supplements may be required for some older people, people with eating disorders, and after some surgical procedures. Low-carbohydrate diets increase the risk of hypoglycaemia when people are taking insulin, sulphonylureas or repaglinide.

Incidence and consequences of malnutrition

The risk of malnutrition increases with increasing age (NHMRC 1999) and probably in people with uncontrolled diabetes. Detecting and managing malnutrition is important because it is associated with increased morbidity and mortality, reduced immunity, and delayed wound healing (Baines and Roberts 2001). In addition, some medications can impair the absorption of essential vitamins and minerals. For example, metformin impairs absorption of vitamin B (Tomkin *et al.* 1971). Iron, zinc, and vitamin C deficiencies are relatively common in older people, and, significantly, people with uncontrolled diabetes may be more deficient in these nutrients than non-diabetics.

Common concomitant conditions that increase the risk of malnutrition in people with diabetes include:

- psychiatric disorders including depression
- Parkinson's disease
- cancer
- HIV/AIDS
- chronic obstructive pulmonary disease
- dental problems
- older and disabled people who are housebound and those with chewing and swallowing difficulties
- polypharmacy, which is common in people with diabetes.

Many people – especially older people in residential care facilities and those who cover up – lack vitamin D and calcium because they are not exposed to sunlight, which increases the risk of osteoporosis, fractures and falls.

It may be difficult and/or impractical for health professionals other than dietitians to undertake comprehensive nutritional assessments, but simple screening tools such as the Nutrition Screening Initiative and Subjective Global Assessment (SGA) can help identify people at risk of poor nutrition and enable appropriate, timely referrals to be made to a dietitian for a comprehensive nutritional assessment and appropriate dietary advice.

Measuring the carbohydrate content of food

A range of methods is used to estimate the carbohydrate content of food. These include:

- portions
- carbohydrate counting
- exchanges
- dose adjustment for normal eating (DAFNE)
- glycaemic index (GI).

Each method has advantages and disadvantages, which need to be considered for the individual (Powers 1996; Brand-Miller *et al.* 1998; International Diabetes Federation (IDF) 2006).

Increasing mobility and exercise

Regular exercise has physical and mental benefits for people with diabetes of all ages. Diet and exercise play a key role in reducing the risk of type 2 diabetes and cardiovascular complications. A recent meta-analysis suggests the benefits of exercise interventions are greater when exercise is the only focus (Conn and Hafdahl 2007). The study also showed that delivering the exercise programme over an extended time achieved better results, and that men reduced their HbA_{1c} and maintained their exercise routines better than women. Significantly, the benefits were the same for those with a high BMI and inadequate metabolic control as for leaner people with good control. However, exercise is difficult for many people, especially older people, because of the decline in muscle mass and so general strength and energy, which increases the risk of falls, injury, and fractures. Aerobic exercise such as Tai Chi for at least 30 minutes/day and strength training exercises such as progressive weightlifting can help maintain muscle mass and energy and have a positive effect on well-being.

CASE DISCUSSION

> **Mr WC**
>
> ***Mr WC self-referred to a diabetes centre at a tertiary hospital***
> I am confused about the recommendations for diet, especially the GI. As a veteran of 27 years of type 1 diabetes, I am also a veteran of a number of treatment schedules, various insulins and diets. The 'one-size-fits-all' approach is inappropriate at best and downright dangerous in some circumstances. I control my blood glucose with long-acting insulin at midnight and rapid-acting insulin before each meal and eating a low GI diet. However, eating low GI foods send my blood glucose down after I eat. When I correct my blood glucose it goes the other way and I get hyperglycaemic because the GI kicks in and so do my recovery hormones.
>   What can I do?

Dietitian

I would seek extra information from his GP about his clinical results (HbA$_{1c}$, lipid profile, blood pressure, BMI) and whether he has any long-term complications such as gastroparesis. In addition, I would clarify the following issues with Mr WC:

- What are his actual blood glucose levels around specific meals and the dietary and medication adjustments he makes to interpret his statement that: 'eating low GI foods sends my blood glucose down after I eat'? Some people feel 'hypo' when their blood glucose levels are above 4 mmol/L. I also need to clarify whether the blood glucose drops after every meal or specific meals or at certain times of the day.
- Does he count carbohydrates? If he does, clarify whether he includes very low GI foods such as pulses and only eats low GI carbohydrates or includes some medium and high GI carbohydrates as well.
- Does he adjust his insulin according to the carbohydrate content of the meal?
- Has he attended any structured/self-management education programmes such as DAFNE?

Once those issues were clarified I would provide the following advice:

- Inform him that the quantity of carbohydrate consumed is the key strategy for optimal glycaemic control and that the quality or GI may only offer additional benefits if the quantity of carbohydrate is considered (Sheard *et al.* 2004).
- If he is only eating low GI foods, I would advise him that his diet may be more nutritionally balanced if he incorporates some medium/high GI carbohydrates into his eating plan.

- I would recommend that he does not count the carbohydrate content of very low GI foods such as pulses.
- Suggest that when he consumes a low GI meal, he experiments with injecting the rapid-acting insulin with the meal or after the meal rather than before it. Carbohydrate digestion and the resultant rise in blood glucose will have commenced before the insulin begins to work.
- If available, offer him the opportunity to attend a structured/self-management education programme to develop the knowledge, skills, and confidence to adjust insulin according to the quantity of carbohydrate consumed.

Diabetes educator

I agree with all the dietitian's strategies, but I would clarify how soon after a meal he tests his blood glucose. He needs to test at least 2 hours after to determine postprandial glucose levels. If he tests sooner he may detect the rise in blood glucose that occurs in the post-absorptive state.

I would also ascertain what long-acting insulin he is using and why he is injecting it at midnight. The type of insulin and injection time may account for some of the variability. I would also check his blood glucose testing equipment and technique and insulin administration technique and injection sites to determine whether they could be a factor. He may be unnecessarily treating hypoglycaemia.

It is not clear whether he exercises and what effect that has on his insulin requirements and timing of meals. Alcohol intake also needs to be considered.

CASE DISCUSSION

> **Mr AT**
>
> ***Mr AT self-referred to the diabetes centre for advice when he was told he needed insulin by his GP***
> I have type 2 diabetes, which is reasonably controlled on Daonil (glibenclamide) but the dose has been gradually increased and the doctor told me I need insulin. I do not want to take insulin. I started on the Atkins diet 4 weeks ago. It is very difficult to stick to but I have lost some weight and my blood glucose now averages about 7 mmol/L. I stopped the Daonil because I had dizzy spells.
> I want to know whether 80 g of carbohydrate a day is enough?

Dietitian

Although some people lose weight and have improved blood glucose control on the Atkins diet and other low-carbohydrate diets, reducing carbohydrates to less than 130 g/day is not recommended for people with diabetes. The long-term consequences are not clear (Sheard *et al.* 2004) and it is very difficult to sustain.

Diabetes educator

Mr AT needs a careful explanation about the progressive nature of type 2 diabetes and the eventual need for insulin (see Chapter 2). The issue needs to be approached with sensitivity – it is very difficult to argue with his personal successful experience (weight loss and reduction in his blood glucose). Sustaining the Atkins programme in the long term may be more difficult. It is important to explore the reasons why he does not want to commence insulin, so that his concerns can be addressed.

The dizzy spells were possibly hypoglycaemia associated with the reduction in carbohydrate. His medicines should be reviewed and he needs advice about how to recognise and manage hypoglycaemia. If he has also commenced an exercise programme he will need advice about avoiding hypoglycaemia during and after exercise (see Chapter 6). It is important that he continues to monitor his blood glucose.

CASE DISCUSSION

> **Mrs POM**
>
> *Mrs POM telephoned the dietitian for advice*
> I am very strict with my diet and do not eat sugary or sweet foods but my blood glucose is always high.
>   Why is that?

Dietitian

Carbohydrate includes both starchy and sugary foods, which are made from glucose. During digestion they break down into glucose, enter the bloodstream, and raise the blood glucose levels. Glucose – not sugar – is the end product of digestion. Sugar is broken down into glucose. People often refer to diabetes as having 'too much sugar' and many health professionals use the term 'blood sugar levels' in an attempt to simplify things for people with diabetes, but the terminology is misleading and confusing.

References

American Diabetes Association (2006) Nutrition recommendations and interventions for diabetes – 2006. A position statement. *Diabetes Care* 29(9): 2140–2157.

Baines S, Roberts D (2001) Undernutrition in the community. *Australian Prescriber* 24(5): 113–115.

Bouchard L, Drapeau V, Provencher V *et al.* (2004) Neuromedin beta: a strong candidate gene linking eating behaviours and susceptibility to obesity. *American Journal of Clinical Nutrition* 80(6): 1478–1486.

Brand-Miller J, Foster-Powell K, Colagiuri S *et al.* (1998) *The GI Factor*. Hodder, Sydney.

Chagnon YC, Perusse L, Weisnagel SJ *et al.* (2000) The human obesity gene map: the 1999 update. *Obesity Research* 8: 89–117.

Conn V, Hafdahl A (2007) Metabolic effects of interventions to increase exercise in adults with type 2 diabetes. *Diabetologia* 50: 913–921.

Egger G (2007) An interview with Professor Gary Egger. Part 1. *Weight Management in Review* 5: 1–4.

Howe M (2007) Weighty issue. *Australian Doctor* 16 March: 43.

International Diabetes Federation (IDF) (2006) Incidence of diabetes. *Diabetes Atlas* 2 (*www.eatlas.idf.org/Incidence/*).

Knowler WC, Barrett-Connor E, Fowler SE *et al.* (Diabetes Prevention Program Research Group) (2002) Reduction in the incidence of type 2 diabetes with lifestyle intervention and metformin. *New England Journal of Medicine* 346: 393–403.

Lindström J, Louheranta A, Mannelin M *et al.* (Finnish Diabetes Prevention Study) (2003) Lifestyle intervention and 3-year results on diet and physical activity. *Diabetes Care* 26(12): 3230–3236.

Marks S (2000) Obesity management. *Current Therapeutics* 41: 6.

Mooradian A, Failla M, Hoogwerf B *et al.* (1994) Selected vitamins and minerals in diabetes care. *Diabetes Care* 17: 464–479.

Moyad M (2007) Fad diets and obesity. Part 1: measuring weight in a clinical setting. *Urology Nursing* 24(2): 114–119.

National Health and Medical Research Council (NHMRC) (1999) *Dietary Guidelines for Older Australians*. NHMRC, Canberra.

Pan XR, Li GW, Hu YH *et al.* (1997) Effects of diet and exercise in preventing NIDDM in people with impaired glucose tolerance. The Da Qing IGT and Diabetes Study. *Diabetes Care* 20: 537–544.

Peterson D, Govindji A (1988) Giving dietary advice to Asian diabetic patients. *Practical Diabetes* 5(7): 683–686.

Powers M (1996) *Handbook of Diabetes Medical Nutrition Therapy*, Chapter 3. Aspen Publishers, Gaithersburg.

Sheard NF, Clark NG, Brand-Miller JC *et al.* (2004) Dietary carbohydrate (amount and type) in the prevention and management of diabetes: a statement by the American Diabetes Association. *Diabetes Care* 27 (9): 2266–2271.

Tomkin G, Hadden D, Weaver J *et al.* (1971) Vitamin B12 status of patients on long-term metformin therapy. *British Medical Journal* 2: 685–687.

Tuomilehto J, Lindström S, Laakso M *et al.* (2001) Finnish Diabetes Prevention Study Group. Prevention of type 2 diabetes mellitus by changes in lifestyle among subjects with impaired glucose tolerance. *New England Journal of Medicine* 344: 1343–1350.

West D (2007) Motivational interviewing improves weight loss in women with type 2 diabetes. *Diabetes Care* 30: 1081–1087.

Recommended reading

American Diabetes Association (2006) Nutrition recommendations and interventions for diabetes – 2006. A position statement. *Diabetes Care* 29(9): 2140–2157.

British Diabetic Association Report (1992) Dietary recommendations for people with diabetes. *Diabetic Medicines* 9: 189–202.

Dietary Guidelines for all Australians (2003) Australian Government Publications, Canberra.

National Health and Medical Research Council (NHMRC) (2003) *Clinical Practice Guidelines for the Management of Overweight and Obesity in Children and Adolescents*. NHMRC, Canberra.

Chapter 5

Pharmacotherapeutic management

Key points

- Medicines should be used in a quality use of medicines framework.
- The medicine regimen should be reviewed regularly, for example as part of routine complication screening, pre- and postoperatively and when stable conditions change.
- Polypharmacy is often necessary to manage the multiple underlying metabolic abnormalities associated with diabetes and its complications and comorbidities.
- Polypharmacy complicates self-management for the person with diabetes and adds to the cost of managing diabetes.
- Concordance with medicines is a complex self-care task that has physical, cognitive, and mental components. Medicines knowledge and social factors also play a role.
- Diet and exercise continue to be essential, even when medicines are needed.

Introduction

Best practice medicine management often entails making complex decisions on the part of prescribers, dispensers and the person administering the medicine – the person with diabetes. Decisions need to be made about the advantages and disadvantages of using medicines for particular individuals considering:

- best practice guidelines
- the availability of objective medicines information (other than pharmaceutical company promotional material)
- safety
- efficacy

- appropriate dose
- dose interval
- cost, including whether to use generic alternatives
- possible contraindications and interactions
- ease of use
- any special instructions for using and monitoring the effects.

Significantly, medicines commonly used to manage diabetes and its complications are among the top 10 medicines associated with medicine-related adverse events, most of which are preventable (Hahn 2007). Insulin is top of the list of medicines misused by patients and those misused by health professionals especially in hospital settings. Other medicines commonly used by people with diabetes in the top 10 include anticoagulants and aspirin (patient misuse) and warfarin and furosemide (health professional misuse). These findings highlight the need for regular comprehensive medicine reviews and patient medicine self-care abilities. They indicate that medicine assessment may be as important as screening for diabetes complications and could contribute to complications.

Effective communication about medicines among health professionals and with the individual is essential to optimal prescribing and medicine self-management by people with diabetes. Inappropriate medicine use contributes to suboptimal outcomes but medicine concordance is a complex issue that encompasses physical and cognitive ability, medicine knowledge, and beliefs and attitudes about medicines (Dunning and Manias 2005; Simpson 2006).

The UK Prospective Diabetes Study (UKPDS) (1993) indicated that only 15% of people with type 2 diabetes maintained acceptable blood glucose control using diet and exercise and required glucose-lowering medicines: many eventually needed insulin. Importantly, health professionals should not delay adding medicines, which is often referred to as intensifying therapy. Managing medicines is an important changing and increasingly complex self-care task for the person with diabetes.

Quality use of medicines

The quality use of medicines (QUM) is a useful framework for appropriately managing medicines and reducing medicine-related adverse events (Pharmaceutical Health and Rational Use of Medicines 2005).

QUM is an holistic risk management approach that recognises medicines are sometimes necessary for primary and secondary prevention and which encompasses:

- using non-medicine options first. Lifestyle modification may be effective initially in type 2 diabetes (see Chapter 4) but insulin is needed from diagnosis in type 1 (see Chapter 2);
- selecting medicines appropriately if medicines are indicated and using them safely and effectively, which encompasses the issues outlined in the first paragraph;
- placing the individual at the centre of care; and
- having systems in place to support effective medicines use such as policies, objective medicines information, and follow-up processes.

Oral hypoglycaemic agents

The major classes of oral hypoglycaemic agents (OHA) target the different metabolic defects associated with type 2 diabetes.

Biguanides reduce insulin resistance and fasting blood glucose. They are the medicine of choice in overweight people with type 2 diabetes unless they are contraindicated; for example, the presence of significant renal, liver, or cardiac disease and possibly alcohol addiction because of the risk of lactic acidosis. Metformin in conjunction with clomiphene may improve fertility in women with polycystic ovarian syndrome (PCOS) but the evidence is conflicting and its role as a treatment for infertility is not clearly defined (Palomba *et al.* 2005). Women with PCOS who are treated with metformin to reduce insulin resistance should probably be informed about the possibility of pregnancy.

Vitamin B12 deficiency is common and under-recognised. It has been reported in the literature intermittently but the impact of potential confounders such as calcium intake and proton pump inhibitor use is often not taken into account. However, increasing duration of metformin use and increasing doses have been shown to contribute to vitamin B12 deficiency (Ting *et al.* 2006). In Ting *et al.*'s study older age was also related to B12 deficiency but the relationship was not clinically significant. Vegetarians were at increased risk and are also at increased risk of folate, vitamin D, iron, calcium and zinc deficiencies. Screening for deficiencies is recommended because it can cause or exacerbate depression, peripheral neuropathy, anaemia, fatigue and dementia (Greenfield 2007).

Secretagogues (sulphonylureas and glitinides) stimulate the beta cells to produce insulin.

Thiazolidinediones (TZD) reduce insulin resistance and daytime preprandial hyperglycaemia and help control fasting blood glucose. Concerns have arisen about the possibility of death associated with rosiglitazone (Nissen and Wolski 2007) but the risk appears to be low. The DREAM (diabetes reduction approaches with ramipril and rosiglitazone medications) study showed the risk of myocardial infarct was 0.6% in the rosiglitazone group versus 0.3% in controls, which was not statistically significantly different. Careful patient assessment before prescribing is warranted and the patient should be fully informed about the risks (Australian Diabetes Society 2007). More definitive information will be available once the RECORD (rosiglitazone evaluated for cardiac outcomes and regulation of glycaemia in diabetes) study, a phase 3 trial to investigate cardiovascular outcomes, is available. There is a risk of congestive heart failure.

The results of the DREAM study suggested rosiglitazone might prevent type 2 diabetes in people with impaired glucose tolerance, but the inconvenience, cost and risk of adverse events outweigh the benefits (Montori *et al.* 2007).

Pioglitazone does not have the same adverse lipid profile (Hughes 2007).

Alpha-glucosidase inhibitors slow carbohydrate digestion and reduce postprandial blood glucose levels (Braddon 2001).

These medicines can be used alone or in combination and they can be effectively combined with insulin. They are not suitable for people with type 1 diabetes who require insulin from diagnosis. Various algorithms for adding OHAs to manage the various metabolic abnormalities that occur in type 2 diabetes have been suggested. For example:

(1) Commence with dietary modification and exercise (see Chapter 4).
(2) Commence a biguanide if HbA_{1c} remains elevated after 3–6 months. Monitor for a further 3 months.
(3) If the HbA_{1c} continues to be high, add a sulphonylurea and monitor for a further 3 months (dual therapy).
(4) If the HbA_{1c} is between 6.5 and 8% after 3 months add a TZD and monitor for 3–6 months (triple therapy). Triple therapy reduces the HbA_{1c} and total daily insulin dose and avoids weight gain (Strowig *et al.* 2004). TZDs take about 3 months to show a therapeutic effect.
(5) If the HbA_{1c} is > 8% using triple therapy, change to two oral agents and insulin (Kuritzky 2006). Combining insulin and metformin reduces insulin resistance and enables a lower dose of insulin to be used and less weight gain (Strowig *et al.* 2004).
(6) The insulin regimen could include: daily, BD, TDS or QID doses depending on individual metabolic parameters, capability, and long-term outlook.

Although triple therapy is safe and effective, the decision to intensify therapy must be made with the patient and after considering all the risks including the complication risk profile. The particular oral agent and/or insulin used depends on the hypoglycaemia risk and potential consequences of hypoglycaemia such as falls (see Chapter 6), the need to control postprandial blood glucose, potential to cause weight gain (sulphonylureas and TZD) and the physiological profile of the medicine.

Table 5.1 shows frequently used OHAs and their common side effects. Blood glucose self-monitoring provides essential information about the effectiveness of the medicines and is used as the basis of day-to-day dose and dose interval adjustment along with the lipid profile and HbA_{1c}. Blood glucose tests are performed before breakfast to monitor fasting glucose levels, and often before other meals, and/or 2 hours after meals, which monitors glucose disposal (clearance).

Combining OHAs and insulin

A combination of insulin and sulphonylureas or biguanides is often used in type 2 diabetes. Usually adding 10–12 units of an intermediate-acting insulin such as Protaphane or a long-acting insulin analogue to the OHA regimen is effective in the first instance. The time of day the insulin is given depends on the blood glucose profile, but it is often administered at bedtime to control the fasting blood glucose level. In addition, it often helps the individual accept the need for insulin by using a staged approach to discontinuing the OHAs.

Continuing metformin helps reduce insulin resistance and reduce the weight gain associated with insulin use (see Chapter 3).

Insulin

Insulin is a hormone secreted by the beta cells of the pancreas, (~0.5–1.0 unit/kg/day) in response to the increase in the blood glucose level after meals. Insulin binds to insulin receptors on cell membranes and facilitates glucose entry into the cell where it is used as fuel (energy) or for storage. Insulin also reduces hepatic glucose production, stimulates fatty acid and amino acid storage and glycogen formation and storage in the liver and skeletal muscle, and limits lipolysis and proteolysis.

If insulin is deficient, protein, fat and carbohydrate metabolism are altered, producing hyperglycaemia and hyperlipidaemia, which increases the risk of short- and long-term diabetes complications.

Table 5.1 Commonly used oral hypoglycaemic medicines, showing their dose range, dose interval and common side effects.

Medicine (generic names)	Proprietary examples	Dose range	Frequency	Duration of action	Metabolised	Common side effects
Sulphonylureas						
Glibenclamide 5 mg	Daonil Euglucon Glimel	2.5–20 mg	Up to 10 mg as a single dose, >10 mg in divided doses Taken with or immediately before food	6–12 h, peak 6–8 h	Liver Kidney (active metabolites)	Weight gain Nausea Anorexia Skin rashes Severe hypoglycaemia, especially in elderly and those with renal dysfunction
Glipizide 5 mg	Minidiab	2.6–40 mg			Liver	Skin reactions Hypoglycaemia (rare)
Gliclazide	Diamicron	Up to 15 mg as a single dose, >15 mg in a twice-daily dose		Up to 24 h, peak 1–3 h		Hypoglycaemia
	Diamicron MR*	30–120 mg	Taken once a day. Dose increments should be 2 weeks apart	Released over 24 h		
Glimepiride	Amaryl	1–4 mg	2–3/day	5–8 h		

Biguanides				
Metformin 500 mg	Diaformin Diabex Glucophage	0.5–1.5 g	May be increased to 3.0 g 1–3 times a day Taken with or immediately after food	Excreted unchanged in urine	Gastrointestinal disturbances Lactic acidosis Hypoglycaemia with other OHAs Reduces vitamin B12 absorption
Glitinides				
Repaglinide Nateglinide	Prandin Starlix	HbA$_{1c}$ < 8% 0.5 mg > 8% 1–2 mg 0.5–16 mg	2–3/day		Hypoglycaemia with other OHAs Weight gain Gastrointestinal disturbance
Thiazolidinediones				
Rosiglitazone Pioglitazone	Avandia Actos	4–8 mg/day 15–30 mg/day			Localised oedema Weight gain CCF Heart failure Raised liver enzymes Pregnancy risk in women with polycystic ovarian disease (Rosiglitazone)
Alpha-glucosidase inhibitors				
Acarbose 25 mg	Glucobay	50–100 mg	TDS with food		GIT problems, e.g. flatulence, diarrhoea Hypoglycaemia

* A sustained release preparation.
OHA, oral glucose-lowering agents; CCF, congestive cardiac failure; GIT, gastrointestinal tract.

A number of different commercial brands of insulin are available, for example Sanofi-Aventis, Novo Nordisk and Eli Lilly. Five main types of insulin are in common use:

Rapid-acting insulin

Rapid-acting insulin should be clear and colourless in appearance. Onset of action is usually within 10 minutes, it peaks at 60 minutes and acts for 24 hours. Examples are lispro (Humalog) and NovoRapid.

Short-acting insulin

Short-acting insulin should be clear and colourless. Examples are Actrapid, Humulin R or Humulin S. They begin to act within 30 minutes, peak in 3–4 hours and continue to act for 6 hours.

Intermediate-acting insulin

These insulins must be mixed gently before they are used and should have a 'skinny milk' appearance after mixing. There are two main types:

(1) Isophane insulin in which the protein protamine is used to slow the insulin absorption rate, e.g. Humulin NPH and Protaphane.
(2) Lente insulin in which zinc is used to slow the absorption, e.g. Humulin L. The onset of action of both types is 2–3 hours, peak 4–10 hours, and the duration of action up to 12–18 hours.

Long-acting insulin

Insulin analogues include Lantus (glargine) and Levemir (detemir). These insulins are colourless, have a fast onset of action and a peakless profile, and act for up to 24 hours. Great care must be taken to ensure long-acting insulin analogues are not confused with short and rapid-acting insulin.

Premixed insulin

Premixed insulins contain short or rapid-acting insulin and a protamine-based intermediate-acting insulin, e.g. NovoMix30, Humulin 20/80, Humalog Mix 25, Mixtard 30/70.

Sliding scales and top-up regimens

Insulin sliding scales are used with insulin infusions during illness, surgical, and day procedures and managing diabetic emergencies (see Chapter 6) but are not advised for routine care, including hospitalised patients. In fact, sliding scales are associated with triple the risk of hyperglycaemia (Queale *et al.* 1997). The origins of the sliding scale are unknown. The term refers to the practice of adjusting the insulin dose according to the immediate blood glucose test result: a reactive step that does not address the reason for the rise in blood glucose, which often goes untreated and hyperglycaemia recurs. Treatment is more effective when insulin is administered prospectively (Hirsch 1997). There are no documented benefits of sliding scales and a prospective randomised trial may help to resolve the question: 'To use or not to use? That is the question.'

A proactive, preventive approach is to increase the dose of or add short-acting insulin to the next prescribed dose of insulin, review the insulin regimen, and make relevant dose and dose interval adjustments for the following and subsequent days. Extra insulin may be required before the next due insulin dose if the blood glucose is > 18 mmol/L and ketones are present during acute intercurrent illness especially in type 1 diabetes. A range of commonly used medicines can affect blood glucose control and need to be considered when interpreting blood glucose profiles (Table 5.2).

Lipid-lowering agents

Medicines as well as diet and exercise are frequently needed to manage lipids, blood pressure, diabetes complications and other comorbidities. Reducing the cardiovascular risk is an important consideration because cardiovascular disease is a common complication unless the blood glucose and lipids can be kept within normal limits. The focus is on reducing cholesterol, especially LDL and triglycerides, and increasing HDL, which facilitates the removal of LDL cholesterol. People with type 2 diabetes and hyperglycaemia often have elevated cholesterol and triglyceride levels and low HDL, which significantly increases the risk of myocardial infarction and acute pancreatitis.

Other cardiovascular risk factors also need to be addressed and are often exacerbated by low HDL levels (Colquhoun 2002). Controlling blood glucose is an important aspect of controlling lipids (Lipid Study Group 1998). Table 5.3 depicts the major classes of lipid-lowering agents. The individual absolute cardiovascular risk profile needs to be considered, rather than the lipid levels alone. Cardiovascular risk factors include age, sex, previous cardiovascular event, current cardiovascular status, presence of hypertension, smoking, and family history of hypercholesterolemia and cardiac disease (see Chapter 7).

Table 5.2 Commonly used medicines that can affect glycaemic control. Many medicines interact with each other. Interactions can become apparent at any stage but particularly when new medicines are added to the regimen, the dose or dose intervals change or the person's health status changes. Interactions range from mild to severe and do not affect everybody taking the medicine. In some cases diabetes may occur as a consequence of medicines.

Medicines that can increase blood glucose	Medicines that can lower blood glucose*
Glucocorticoids affect catecholamine hormone production and cause insulin resistance. In high doses they affect beta cell function	Non-selective beta blockers such as propanolol, which can delay recovery from hypoglycaemia and/or mask the symptoms
Atypical antipsychotics such as clozapine	Aspirin
Diuretics, especially thiazides	Cyclosporin
Oestrogen preparations	Renally excreted aminoglycosides
Some protease inhibitors used to treat HIV infection, such as indinavar	
Growth hormone used for body building	Alcohol
Over the counter medicines containing sugar and adrenaline	

* These can induce or inhibit liver enzymes or affect renal excretion.

Glucosamine, which is a frequently used complementary medicine to manage arthritic conditions, does not cause hyperglycaemia. It is not recommended if people have an allergy to shellfish.

Compiled from Shenfield (2006)

Antihypertensive agents

Non-medicine treatment of hypertension should be part of the diabetes management plan and should continue even when antihypertensive agents are required. Treatment may include:

- **weight management,** by reducing the amount of fat, alcohol, salt, and sweet foods in the diet and increasing the amount of fruit, vegetables, and wholegrain cereal (see Chapter 4);
- **regular exercise** where possible, for example, walking and swimming, which help control weight and increase cardiovascular fitness;

Table 5.3 Commonly used lipid-lowering agents.

Lipid-lowering drug	Main action	Management considerations
HMG-CoA reductase inhibitors	Reduce LDL-c	Test liver function on commencing and in 6 months
		Use caution if liver disease is present
		Decrease the dose if the patient commences cyclosporine
Fibrates	Reduce cholesterol and triglycerides and increase HDL-c	Can be combined with HMG-CoA after a trial on monotherapy
		Monitor creatinine kinase and liver function at 6 weeks and then in 6 months
		May cause GIT disturbances
Resins (cholestyramine, colestipol)	Enhance LDL-c lowering effects of HMG-CoA agents	Allows lower doses of the resins to be used
		Slows absorption of oral hypoglycaemic agents and increases hypoglycaemia risk when used with these agents
Low-dose nicotinic acid		Can be given with HMG-CoA agents
		Enhances reduction of triglyceride and HDL-c
Statins	Reduce LDL-c	Can be used with a resin
	Have a moderate effect on triglycerides	Monitor liver function
	Increase HDL	May cause myositis
	Increase bone mineral density	

- **stress management** considering the individual's preference and capability, for example Tai Chi, meditation, relaxation classes; and
- **stop smoking,** if necessary through quit programmes.

A stepwise approach to controlling hypertension is usually recommended to achieve blood pressure targets (National Heart Foundation of Australia 2001; World Health Organization/International Society for Hypertension Guidelines 2003).

(1) Establish baseline blood pressure risk factor profile and presence of other diabetes complications and comorbidities. Undertaking 24-hour ambulatory blood pressure monitoring may be helpful to distinguish between sustained hypertension and 'white coat' hypertension.

(2) Exclude secondary causes of hypertension such as endocrine diseases, e.g. hyperaldosteronism, Cushing's syndrome, renal artery stenosis or medicine-induced hypertension, including complementary medicines such as liquorice. Analgesic use may be associated with hypertension in people with normal blood pressure. For example, paracetamol use was associated with increases in blood pressure in 34% of 16 031 males after 6–7 weeks of regular use. While the results of this study may not be generalisable, many people with diabetes have concomitant diseases and complications that cause pain and use these medicines. Non-medicines options and complementary therapies such as acupuncture and massage may be useful alternatives or enable lower doses of analgesics to be used (see Chapter 11).

(3) Determine baseline blood lipids, electrolytes, urea, creatinine, urinary albumin excretion rate, cardiac status, ECG or echocardiography.

(4) Modify lifestyle behaviours that increase risk such as diet, exercise and smoking.

(5) Introduce antihypertensive agents as indicated (Table 5.4).

Salicylates

Salicylates, for example aspirin, clopidogrel, Persantin (dipyridamole) and ticlopidine, are indicated to prevent platelet aggregation in people with type 2 diabetes over 45 years who have cardiovascular risk factors, if lifestyle modification is ineffective. Regular monitoring to detect bleeding is important and might occur if anticoagulants and some complementary medicines are used concomitantly (see Chapter 11). Bruising may also occur at injection sites.

Recent analysis of a subset of patients in the GeneStar study ($n = 139$) who did not comply with directions to avoid foods such as grapefruit, caffeine-containing foods, wine, cocoa-containing foods, and chocolate suggests dark chocolate has similar antithrombotic effects to aspirin (Faraday 2006). Chocolate inhibits platelet activation regardless of age, gender, BMI, systolic blood pressure, cholesterol, fibrinogen and Von Willebrand factor. However, the effects are small and there may be other unwanted effects such as weight gain.

Table 5.4 Indications for and potential adverse events associated with commonly prescribed antihypertensive agents.

Antihypertensive agent	Examples	Indications	Potential adverse effects
Angiotensin-converting enzyme (ACE) inhibitors These medicines improve cardiac remodelling and stabilise the rate of progression of renal disease	Monopril (fosinopril) Coversyl (perindopril) Accupril (quinapril) Gopten (trandolalpril)	Heart failure Previous cardiac event Microalbuminuria	Hypotension with the first dose Hyperkalaemia Angioedema Cough, which can become irritating to others Renal impairment if renal disease is present
Angiotensin receptor antagonists	Telmisartan Candesartan Losartan	Albuminuria Heart failure Previous cardiac event ACE inhibitor not tolerated	Hypotension with first dose Reduced glomerular filtration rate Hyperkalaemia Rarely angioedema and persistent cough Renal impairment if renal disease is present
Beta-blocking agents (cardioselective agents preferred)	Atenolol Metroprolol	Heart failure Previous cardiac event	Hypo- or hyperglycaemia Hypoglycaemic unawareness Worse peripheral vascular disease Erectile dysfunction Depression Sleep disturbance
Calcium channel blocking agents: centrally acting and peripherally acting vasodilators	Amlodipine Nifedpine Diltiazem Verapamil		Gastrointestinal effects such as constipation, oesophageal reflux especially with centrally acting Flushing Headache Peripheral oedema
Diuretics, e.g. low-dose thiazides	Aprinox (bendroflumethiazide) Hygroton (chlortalidone)	Symptomatic heart failure	Hyperglycaemia Hyperkalaemia Hyponatraemia Dyslipidaemia Hyperuraemia Erectile dysfunction
Sympatholytics, e.g. not with beta blocker	Aldomet (methyldopa) Hydopa (methyldopa) Catapres (clonidine)		Depression Postural hypotension

Reproduced with permission from Dunning T (2003) *Care of People with Diabetes*. Blackwell Publishing, Oxford.

CASE DISCUSSION

Mr KM

Mr KM was referred to a tertiary diabetes centre by his GP
Mr KM is a 77-year-old man who has had type 2 diabetes for 17 years.
  Current HbA$_{1c}$ 9.5%
  Random blood glucose 24 mmol/L
  Hyperlipidaemia
  BP 165/70
  Retinopathy proliferative
  Renal dysfunction
  Cardiomyopathy and past history AMI and stent
  Pacemaker in place

Current medications
Daonil (glibenclamide)	10 mg	BD
Jezil (gemfibrozil)	150 mg	daily
Karvea (irbesartan)	150 mg	daily
Protaphane	24 units mane, 20 units nocte	
Clopidogrel	75 mg	daily
Sotalol	40 mg	BD
Irbesartan	150 mg	
Frusemide		

Referred to commence metformin.
  Very tired and not sleeping.
  Wife is very unwell in a nursing home. Mr KM visits her each day and spends the day holding her hand 'which keeps her calm and helps her sleep' and mostly sleeps sitting beside her.

Diabetes educator

Mr KM highlights the importance of considering the individual's specific circumstances and life priorities and not just his diabetes status. Importantly it highlights the key role of family support in managing diabetes and the need to consider the family as well as the person with diabetes. Being tired and sleeping poorly is most likely a combination of stress and anxiety generated by having his wife in a nursing home. This is likely to contribute to his hyperglycaemia, which increases his tiredness, setting up a vicious cycle. Having said that, the majority of people with long standing diabetes and poor glycaemic control have an inadequate medication regimen.

Mr KM could be depressed. Depression is an under-diagnosed complication of diabetes. Goldney *et al.* (2004) found that approximately

1 in 4 people with diabetes are depressed. Reynolds (1999) found a correlation between chronic conditions and major depression in older people. A mental health assessment would be very useful to determine Mr KM's level of stress, anxiety and depression and devise strategies to help him cope. Suggesting his GP coordinates a management plan that may or may not involve medication may facilitate such a consultation. His cognitive status could also be assessed.

It would be helpful to review Mr KM's diet. He may be neglecting his diet since his wife was placed in a nursing home, and is at significant risk of malnutrition. It may be possible for the nursing home to provide him with a meal during his daily visits. It is not uncommon for family members who visit residential care facilities on a daily basis to be encouraged to have a greater role in caring for their loved ones, which may reduce their feeling of helplessness but can also be a burden. There may be activities that Mr KM and his wife could enjoy together that involve more than holding hands and sleeping all day, which probably contributes to Mr KM's inability to sleep well at night.

The hyperglycaemia does need to be addressed and has been present for at least 3 months judging by the HbA_{1c}. The possibility of reduced medication compliance especially during this period of profound stress needs to be considered. A structured medication review is indicated to find a way to simplify his medicine regimen.

Metformin may be contraindicated. Mr KM has renal dysfunction, although the degree of damage is not clear from the referral history and needs to be clarified. Renal failure is a contraindication to metformin because of the possibility of lactic acidosis, which is fatal in approximately 50% of cases. His age and high risk of becoming dehydrated are also contraindications to metformin, for the same reason. He is using two antihypertensive agents from the same class and this needs to be revised.

Long-acting sulphonylureas such as Daonil (glibenclamide) may not be the best choice in an older person because it has a long half-life, increasing the risk of hypoglycaemia, which he may not recognise. Mr KM's renal impairment also increases the risk of hypoglycaemia. This point is often forgotten when HbA_{1c} is the prime focus. Hypoglycaemia can still occur despite an HbA_{1c} of 9.5% if the food intake is poor, and in an older person with impaired renal functioning it can be prolonged and severe.

A TZD could be considered depending on the degree of heart failure and could help maintain the patency of his stent. Agents such as Avandia (rosiglitazone) and Actos (pioglitazone) can be prescribed in people with diabetes with Class 1 and 2 heart failure defined by the New York Heart Association. Careful monitoring of liver function (transaminase levels) and fluid retention is required. TZDs generally take at least 3 months to show therapeutic benefit. However, given that Mr KM also has cardiomyopathy I would not use a TZD.

An alpha-glucosidase inhibitor could be considered. Acarbose prolongs the time it takes for food to be absorbed, thereby reducing postprandial blood glucose excursions. However, it is often associated with intolerable gastrointestinal tract side effects. Generally, acarbose only reduces HbA_{1c} by 0.5% and adding an additional tablet that must be taken after food would complicate his medicine regimen at a very stressful time. Although acarbose does not cause hypoglycaemia, the other OHAs might, in which case hypoglycaemia must be treated with glucose because acarbose inhibits sucrose absorption.

Protaphane has a variable action profile and changing to a long-acting insulin analogue might reduce the complexity of his medication regimen. Rapid-acting insulin may also be needed at meal times. Possible strategies include:

- Cease Protaphane and switch to twice-daily Levemir (detemir).
- Cease Protaphane and switch to daily Lantus (glargine).
- Cease Protaphane and change to twice-daily premixed insulin such as NovoMix30 or HumalogMix25 because the rapid-acting component is less likely to cause mid-morning and pre-bed hypoglycaemia compared with Mixtard 30/70 or Humulin 30/70 whose fast-acting component peaks at approximately 4 hours (and therefore often late morning or at bedtime).
- Cease Daonil (glibenclamide) and commence Diamicron MR (modified-release gliclazide) 120 mg with breakfast. This long-acting 24-hour agent is activated when blood glucose levels rise. Alternatively, the oral agents could be ceased altogether, which would simplify the medicine regimen.

In addition, I would check Mr KM's insulin administration technique and the type of insulin delivery device he is using. He has proliferative retinopathy and may not be able to see to dial up the correct insulin dose or the device. According to Sinclair and Finucane (2001), 10% of older people with diabetes have sight-threatening retinopathy. Protaphane is dispensed in a variety of devices. If his insulin was dispensed in a different device from usual Mr KM might be confused about how to use the device. The InnoLet is often easier for older people to use because the numbers are large and dialling up is relatively easy because the device looks like an egg timer. Depressing the plunger to deliver the insulin does not require as much strength or dexterity as some other devices. The drawback is the limited range of insulins available in the InnoLet.

I would also check his insulin administration sites to assess whether he has any hypertrophy, which could affect insulin absorption. Mr KM's blood glucose testing technique also needs to be assessed. He may not be testing because of the stress and worry associated with his wife's condition and may not see his health as a priority while his wife is unwell. This is an important issue to identify. Often when a spouse is unwell, the partner neglects his or her own health needs. Mr KM needs to be aware that he needs to care for himself to be strong and well enough to assist his wife. He may need support to do so.

I would also like to exclude asymptomatic angina. Mr KM has had one MI and his stent may no longer be patent. Asymptomatic angina is common in people with diabetes. An estimated one in five AMIs occur without symptoms in this population. Measuring his creatine kinase (CK) and an ECG would be useful.

Other issues to consider:

- Fibrates (Jezil, gemfibrozil) are contraindicated in severe renal impairment and may need to be reviewed once the degree of renal impairment is established.
- Mr KM is prescribed both Karvea (proprietary name) and ibesartan (generic name): both are angiotensin-II antagonists. Insomnia is an infrequent side effect of the angiotensin-II antagonists. Mr KM is taking two of these agents, which could contribute to his difficulty sleeping.
- An additional consideration related to his poor sleeping patterns is obstructive sleep apnoea (OSA). If it is not diagnosed and treated, OSA results in a very poor sleep during the night and the necessary deep sleep and relaxation are compromised.

Diabetes educator 2

I agree with this comprehensive assessment. Treatment decisions in older people with diabetes are complicated by many factors including health status and life expectancy. Many older people express a desire to maintain their independence, and avoiding the burden of complex self-care and medicine regimens is often valued over longevity. Mr KM's desires in this respect may influence his management. He has considerable health risks, which will also influence the management. Controlling lipids and hypertension may confer greater benefits than controlling blood glucose (Durso 2006).

There is evidence that daily glargine in combination with oral glucose-lowering agents simplifies the medicine regimen and achieves acceptable blood glucose control with a lower risk of hypoglycaemia in older people (Janka *et al.* 2005).

Endocrinologist

This gentleman needs excellent control. Metformin is contraindicated because of the renal insufficiency and adding a glitazone would be my choice, possibly with a long-acting insulin analogue.

CASE DISCUSSION

Mrs RS

Mrs RS was referred to an endocrinologist by her GP
Mrs RS is a 60-year-old woman with type 2 diabetes. She has a strong family history of hypercholestaemia, hypertension and cardiac disease. She smokes 10–12 cigarettes per day and had CAGS (coronary artery bypass grafts) 2 years ago.
 Her HbA$_{1c}$ is 9.6% and she is obese.
 She has xanthomata on her hands and lipaemia retinalis.

Current medications
Metformin	2 g	BD
Gliclazide	240 mg	daily
Gemfibrosil		
Aspirin		
Atorvastatin	80 mg	daily
Amlodipine		
Valsartan		

The dietitian told her to try harder with her diet and do more exercise and the diabetes educator told her to stop smoking.
 Most things seem to be reasonably controlled, but she is complaining of aching joints.
 Please assess and advise.

Podiatrist

Mrs RS' feet need to be assessed to rule out peripheral neuropathy and arterial disease before Mrs RS starts walking, which like other weight-bearing exercises is not recommended if these conditions are present. Alternatives include non-weightbearing exercise such as using an exercise bike, swimming, or upper body exercises. I would suggest she consults an exercise physiologist or physiotherapist experienced in managing chronic diseases who could advise about a safe exercise programme.

A podiatrist could advise about appropriate footwear and pain management if the aching joints include her feet. Obese people often suffer from foot pain, commonly through injury to the plantar fascia (arch). The podiatrist could recommend stretches. Modify her footwear, for example by providing inner soles, or local strapping of the feet.

Diabetes educator

The last statement on the referral: '*Most things seem to be reasonably controlled . . .*' is belied by Mrs RS' obesity, HbA_{1c}, complication status, and probably lipid levels, which were not provided, but are likely to be high given the lipaemia retinalis and xanthoma. I would refer her to an endocrinologist for a thorough review, especially her lipid medications and OHA regimen. Statins may be contraindicated, depending on her lipid profile. She may have some renal impairment given her cardiovascular status. Considering her HbA_{1c} and lipidaemia she probably needs insulin. Gliclazide contributes to weight gain. Metformin might be contraindicated due to her cardiac status. In the first instance she might benefit from a short admission and an intravenous insulin infusion to reduce her lipid levels. She is at risk of acute pancreatitis as well as a cardiovascular event.

A thorough pain assessment is indicated. Statins are known to cause myalgia and contribute to aching joints and this is a possible cause of her problem. Alternatively, her weight may contribute to her joint pain. People often stop taking statins because of aching joints. The possibility that Mrs RS is having a silent MI should be investigated (ECG, troponins, cardiac enzymes) depending on the location of the pain and its onset and duration. Some of the weight gain could also be due to oedema as a result of her cardiac status.

Given Mrs RS' lipid status, it would be important to tactfully establish whether she is taking her medicines. Bone density studies might be indicated given her obesity, age, and smoking habit, to determine whether she has an osteoporotic fracture.

Mrs RS has probably been repeatedly 'nagged' about her health status. A different approach is needed, for example discussing her life and health goals. Exercise may be difficult given her obesity and cardiac status. Cardiac rehabilitation or Tai Chi might be beneficial. An appropriate diet is essential but creative ways of providing dietary advice need to be devised and should consider her living arrangements, ability to shop and cook, financial status and nutritional status. She is probably malnourished despite her obesity.

She needs to stop smoking. She may be able to reduce or stop smoking if she was referred to a quit programme. However, stopping smoking might contribute to weight gain and could be one reason she has not stopped. Psychological counselling might be beneficial if she agrees.

Endocrinologist

This woman should stop smoking. In addition she has lipaemia retinalis, which suggests very severe hyperlipidaemia, possibly type 3. She needs apolipoprotein E and lipoprotein electrophoresis to evaluate whether she has severe hypertriglyceridemia. If so, statin therapy would be contraindicated and fenofibrate plus fish oil and possibly even nicotinic acid therapy may be needed.

CASE DISCUSSION

Mr VR

Mr VR was referred to the endocrinology department of a major hospital to 'get his diabetes fixed up' after he presented to the emergency department
Mr VR is a 69-year-old man with type 2 diabetes of many years' duration.

He has high postprandial blood glucose levels in the morning – up to 16 mmol/L from ~7 mmol/L and before tea up to 10 mmol/L.

Current medications

Diabex (metformin)	2 mg	TDS
Diamicron (gliclazide)	1 mg	BD
Actos (pioglitazone)	30 mg	mane
Anpec (verapamil)	⎫	
Astrix (aspirin)	⎬ dose not specified	
Coversyl (perindopril)	⎭	

He has nocturia, which is disturbing his sleep.

His Diamicron was increased to the above dose to improve the problem of postprandial hyperglycaemia and nocturia with no effect.

What do I do now?

General practitioner

Mr VR has several issues. These include nocturia that could be related to Actos (pioglitazone), which causes fluid retention and hyperglycaemia, or prostate problems. He has both fasting and post-prandial hyperglycaemia that has not improved despite increasing his OHA doses. I would like to know his HbA_{1c}. I would check the basics to assess whether Mr VR is eating appropriately and is suitably active.

The first consideration is to ensure that Mr VR is taking all his medications appropriately. In a survey performed by Ultrafeedback, fewer than three in four patients said they always took medication as directed; 23% admitted they sometimes forgot to do so, and 4% said they generally did not take prescribed medications at all. There are many reasons for these findings such as cost, the number of tablets, knowledge about the medication, and age. People should be asked about their medication use in a non-judgmental manner. Assessing medication self-management is an important aspect of managing chronic illnesses such as diabetes.

Mr VR needs a medication review that can be undertaken by his doctor, or a formal medication review could be undertaken by a pharmacist through the home medication review (HMR) programme to help determine his medication self-management practices and improve his understanding of – and compliance with – medication. Involving pharmacists in medication management can lead to reductions in HbA_{1c} of ~ 1%.

Increasing his OHA doses is worthwhile because he is not on maximal doses of Diamicron (gliclazide). Reducing his metformin dose to 1 mg BD should be considered because compliance with TDS dosing is usually poor and the side effects of 2 mg TDS could be contributing to non-compliance.

Mr VR's nocturia needs to be assessed by taking a full history and relevant investigations, including a prostate check. Assuming that the nocturia is not related to prostate disease, fluid retention from Actos should be considered, as well as nocturnal hyperglycaemia. With a fasting glucose of 7 mmol/L, fluid retention is likely to be the cause of the nocturia. Controlling the glucose levels overall is a good first line strategy. If that does not improve Mr VR's nocturia, consideration should be given to stopping Actos, especially if he has significant fluid retention and peripheral oedema.

The strength of primary care is the ability to have timely reviews of patients especially when the diagnosis is not clear.

Diabetes educator

The GP has addressed the important considerations. I would also assess Mr VR's blood glucose testing technique to determine how long after food he waits before testing his blood glucose. If he is testing soon after a meal, he may be recording post-absorptive glucose levels, which are likely to be higher than postprandial levels measured 2 hours after food. He may need a diet and exercise review.

The possibility of silent urinary tract infection needs to be considered and a microurine and culture is indicated. Nocturia disrupts sleep and reduces quality of life.

CASE DISCUSSION

Mr TRE

Mr TRE was referred to an endocrinologist by his GP
I am not sure how to manage this 70-year-old man.

He has a strong family history of diabetes and was diagnosed 2 years ago, when he had minor surgery after he fractured his arm falling off a ladder while cleaning out his gutters. His blood glucose was 22 mmol/L postoperatively and he was commenced on Daonil (glibenclamide).

Since then he has continued to lose weight and is very tired. His HbA$_{1c}$ is 11% and most of his blood tests are high. I increased the Daonil but it does not seem to help.

Do you think I should start insulin?

General practitioner and diabetes educator

We need to determine whether Mr TRE has type 1 or type 2 diabetes (see Chapter 2). I would test his C-peptide levels, GAD (glutamic acid decarboxylase) and IA$_2$ antibodies and undertake a full clinical assessment. I think he needs insulin and a full medication review. If insulin were started, he would benefit from a dietitian review.

His social circumstances, understanding of diabetes, and the presence of symptoms need to be established. The weight loss is probably due to hyperglycaemia but other causes such as cancer and thyroid disease need to be considered. He may be malnourished and at risk of osteoporosis. In addition, his mental status could be compromised by the hyperglycaemia, which is likely to affect his self-care capacity and put him at risk of hyperosmolar states and falls.

CASE DISCUSSION

Mr BG

Mr BG was referred to a diabetes multidisciplinary team by his GP

Mr BG is a 70-year-old man. Can you help me develop an appropriate management plan? He has had diabetes since 1999. His presenting problem is a chronic cough and haemoptysis and sleep apnoea.

He has a long history of a series of illnesses and surgical interventions including prostate cancer, renal calculi and minor infections such as tinea. He appears to be atopic with a history of skin allergies, hay fever and conjunctivitis.

He has irritable bowel syndrome and eats a gluten-free diet.

Diabetes complications include peripheral neuropathy and cardiovascular disease.

He has regular acupuncture for osteoarthritis in his knees.

Current medications

Amaryl (glimepiride)	1 mg	daily with first main meal of day. With half a glass of water.
Atacand Plus 16/12.5 tablets (candesartan cilexetil)	16 mg/12.5 mg	1 daily
Co-enzyme Q10 capsule	100 mg	1 daily with food
Coversyl tablet – ceased (perindopril)	8 mg	1 daily
Diprosone lotion (betamethasone)	0.05%	BD pm
Ditropan tablet (oxybutynin)	5 mg	1 TID
Iscover tablet (clopidogrel)	75 mg	1 daily
Metformin hydrochloride tablet	500 mg	2 BD
Nexium tablet (esomeprazole)	20 mg	1 daily
Norvasc tablet (amlodipine)	10 mg	1 mane
Rhinocort (budesonide)	dose and dose frequency not indicated	
Seretide (fluticasone)		

His current HbA$_{1c}$	6.5%
Microalbuminuria	'stable' (no values provided)
Cholesterol	3.6 mmol/L
LDL	2.0 mmol/L
HDL	1.0 mmol/L
Triglycerides	1.4 mmol/L

His blood pressure is stable at present and he had a recent weight loss of 4–5 kg since consulting a naturopath.

General practitioner

Mr BG has a long history of a series of illnesses and surgical interventions including prostate cancer, renal calculi, and minor infections such as tinea. He appears to be atopic with a history of skin allergies, hay fever, and conjunctivitis. He has irritable bowel syndrome and eats a gluten-free diet.

Diabetes complications include peripheral neuropathy and cardiovascular disease. He has regular acupuncture for osteoarthritis in his knees. His blood pressure is reported to be stable at present but no specific information about his levels was provided. He had a recent weight loss of 4–5 kg since consulting a naturopath but we have no information about his weight status. He appears to have good control with an HbA_{1c} of 6.5% but he has haemoptysis. However, this may not be a true reflection of his metabolic control (see Chapter 2) and serum fructosamine could be considered.

The most important issue is to investigate and manage the haemoptysis and chronic cough as a matter of urgency. The weight loss adds an ominous aspect to the case study. Cancer of the lung needs to be excluded and then other causes such as TB. Initially, a chest X-ray and sputum cytology/microculture and acid fast testing should be performed.

If radioactive dyes are needed for any radiological interventions he will need to cease his metformin two days before the investigation and will need written advice about that. His renal function needs to be assessed to determine whether it is safe to continue metformin. The estimated glomerular filtration rate (eGFR) should be calculated rather than relying on the creatinine level alone (see Chapter 3).

Metformin may be causing his 'irritable bowel' or aggravating his symptoms. Alternatively, the symptoms may be related to autonomic neuropathy, which often causes bloating, vomiting, diarrhoea and fluctuating blood glucose levels.

If surgery is required, temporarily using insulin to control his glucose levels through surgery and in the immediate postoperative phase leads to better outcomes and makes management easier. If chemotherapy is required, it can have various effects on Mr BG's blood glucose levels, depending on the chemotherapeutic agents used. Commencing insulin – especially if the blood glucose is erratic – can simplify the medicine regimen and make the blood glucose easier to control. The blood glucose can be affected by the chemotherapy agents (e.g. corticosteroids) as well as nausea and not eating.

Heart disease is the most common cause of death in people with diabetes. The lipid profile suggests he is already taking a statin, which, considering his vascular disease, neuropathy, nephropathy, prostate cancer, as well as his age, puts Mr BP as a likely candidate for surgery.

Diabetes educator

The GP raised very important issues but did not appear to consider the implications of the weight loss following Mr BG's consultation with a naturopath. The weight loss may be inappropriate and related to cancer, as the GP suggested. However, it may be appropriate and improve his osteoarthritis and cardiovascular status. It would be important to determine why he consulted the naturopath and what, if anything, the naturopath prescribed. Mr BG also uses acupuncture to manage osteoarthritic pain. It is important to establish whether the acupuncturist uses sterile technique, which is likely in most developed countries but not always the case in other places.

His use of complementary therapies indicates he actively participates in self-care and is proactive. The GP referred Mr BG for advice about developing a care plan. It would be essential to include his complementary therapy practitioners in such planning and to ensure his complementary treatments are documented in the conventional medical record (see Chapter 11). Complementary medicine interactions and contraindications may need to be considered as part of the medicine review.

Probiotics may help with his gastrointestinal tract symptoms by encouraging beneficial intestinal flora and reducing fermentation of undigested food, which accumulates due to gastric stasis. Likewise, peppermint oil enteric-coated capsules in low doses may help with his gastrointestinal symptoms provided he does not have oesophageal reflux or gall bladder disorders (Kligler and Chaudhary 2007).

He may have foot pathology as a consequence of the tinea, which needs to be assessed. In addition his ability to care for his feet may be compromised by his osteoarthritis and possibly retinopathy or blurred vision due to hyperglycaemia. I would refer him to a podiatrist for foot assessment and education. Charcot's arthropathy needs to be excluded, or managed if it is present. The extent of the tinea should be assessed. For example he may have tinea in skin folds that also needs to be treated and he could have intestinal *Candida* given his atopic history.

I would consider an alternative to Amaryl (glimepiride) given his atopic status. Skin rashes are a known but uncommon side effect of sulphonylureas and Amaryl could be contributing to his skin problems.

If Mr BG does have cancer or TB, he and his family will need appropriate counselling and help making difficult life decisions about treatment options, advanced directives, and making a will.

Podiatrist

The presence of both peripheral neuropathy and tinea pedis puts this man at high risk of foot ulceration. Once the skin integrity is affected by tinea, secondary bacterial infection can rapidly progress to ulceration and cellulitis particularly given his hyperglycaemia, which impairs the immune response. Tinea is a common cause of cellulitis in people with diabetes.

Preventive foot care is essential, although it may not be the priority in this man. Foot hygiene needs to be assessed. He may need education about washing his feet in a pH-neutral product or soap-free skin wash, which is preferable, given his atopic history. He should be advised not to soak his feet, which can cause maceration and increases the risk of infection.

After cleaning his feet he needs to dry them thoroughly, particularly between the toes where the tinea is likely to be. He should change his socks daily. Topical fungicide lotions and creams such as terbinafine, rather than powders, are recommended and may need to be continued for 1–2 weeks after visible signs of infection subside.

Preventing reinfection is important. As well as foot hygiene he should alternate his shoes and not wear the same pair every day. He could wash his socks (and possibly underwear) in an antifungal rinse available from the supermarket and dry them in the sun.

He needs to be educated about the implications of his neuropathy. Intensive foot education, assessing his daily foot care practices and treating any small injuries are essential. A podiatrist can advise about and manage abnormal foot shape such as clawed toes.

CASE DISCUSSION

> **Mr POL**
>
> *Mr POL telephoned to ask when he should take his Diamicron and metformin tablets because 'everybody tells me something different'*

Dietitian

It is probably best to take your Diamicron (gliclazide) with your meal, but you can take it 30 minutes before you eat. However, if your meal is delayed, your blood glucose could go too low. Metformin can cause gastric upsets, so it is best to take it with food.

References

Australian Diabetes Society (ADS) (2007) *A Position Statement on Rosiglitazone (Avandia®)*. ADS, Sydney.

Braddon J (2001) Oral hypoglycaemics: a guide to selection. *Current Therapeutics* Suppl 13: 42–47.

Colquhoun DM (2002) Lipid-lowering agents. *Australian Family Physician* 31(1): 25–30.

Dunning T (2003) *Care of People with Diabetes*. Blackwell Publishing, Oxford.

Dunning, T, Manias E (2005) Medication knowledge and self-management by people with type 2 diabetes. *Australian Journal of Advanced Nursing* 11: 172–181.

Durso S (2006) Using clinical guidelines designed for older adults with diabetes mellitus and complex health status. *Journal of the American Medical Association* 295: 1935–1940.

Faraday N (2006) *Chocolate Has Antithrombotic Effects Similar to Aspirin*. Proceedings of the American Heart Association Scientific Sessions, Abstract 4101, 14 November.

Goldney R, Phillips P, and Fisher L (2004) Diabetes, depression and quality of life. *Diabetes Care* 27: 1066–1070.

Greenfield R (2007) Oh, to B12 again . . . metformin use and B12 deficiency. *Alternative Medicine Alert* 10(4): 46–47.

Hahn K (2007) *The 'Top 10' Drug Errors and How to Prevent Them*. Proceedings of the American Pharmacists Association Annual Meeting, Atlanta, March.

Hirsch I (1997) Sliding scale insulin in hospitalised patients. Summary and comment. *International Diabetes Monitor* 9(5): 14–15.

Hughes S (2007) The rosiglitazone aftermath: legitimate concerns or hype? *Medscape News* (*www.medscape.com/viewarticle/557198*).

Janka H, Plewe G, Busch K (2005) Combination of oral antidiabetic agents with basal insulin versus premixed insulin alone in randomized elderly patients with type 2 diabetes. Proceedings of the American Diabetes Association Scientific Sessions, Abstract 583-P.

Kligler B, Chaudhary S (2007) Peppermint oil may relieve digestive symptoms and headaches. *American Family Physician* 75: 1027–1030.

Kuritzky L (2006) Addition of basal insulin to oral antidiabetic agents: a goal-directed approach to type 2 diabetes therapy. *Medscape General Medicine* 6(4): 34–47.

Lipid Study Group (1998) The long-term intervention with pravastatin in ischaemic disease. Prevention of cardiovascular events and death with pravastatin in patients with coronary heart disease and a broad range of initial cholesterol levels. *New England Journal of Medicine* 339: 1349–1357.

Montori VM, Isley WL, Guyatt GH (2007) Waking from the DREAM of preventing diabetes with drugs. *British Medical Journal* 334: 882–884.

National Heart Foundation (2001) *Lipid Management Guidelines.* National Heart Foundation, Melbourne.

Nissen SE, Wolski K (2007) Effect of rosiglitazone on the risk of myocardial infarction and death from cardiovascular causes. *New England Journal of Medicine* 356(24): 2457–2471.

Palomba S, Orio F Jr, Falbo A *et al.* (2005) Prospective parallel randomised double-blind, double-dummy controlled clinical trial comparing clomiphene citrate and metformin as the first line treatment for ovulatory induction in non-obese women with polycystic ovary syndrome. *Journal of Clinical Endocrinology and Metabolism* 90: 4068–4074.

Pharmaceutical Health and Rational Use of Medicines Committee (2005) *The Quality Use of Medicines in Diabetes.* Department of Health and Ageing, Canberra.

Phillips PJ, Popplewell P, Wing L (2003) Diabetes and hypertension – double trouble. *Medicine Today*, 1–9.

Queale W, Seidler A, Brancati F (1997) Glycemic control and sliding scale insulin use in medical inpatients with diabetes mellitus. *Archives of Internal Medicine* 157: 545–552.

Reynolds C (1999) Depression and ageing: a look to the future. *Psychiatry Service* 50: 1167–1172.

Shenfield G (2006) Common medicines that may affect glycaemic stability. *Diabetes Management Journal* 17: 28–29.

Simpson R (2006) Challenges of improving medication adherence. *Journal of the American Medical Association (http://jama.amaassn. org/cgi/content/full/296.21.jed60074v1).*

Sinclair J, Finucane P (2001) *Diabetes in Old Age.* John Wiley and Sons, Chichester.

Strowig S, Aviles-Santa M, Raskin P (2004) Improved glycaemic control without weight gain using triple therapy in type 2 diabetes. *Diabetes Care* 27: 1577–1563.

Ting RZ, Szeto CC, Chan MH *et al.* (2006) Risk factors of vitamin B12 deficiency in patients receiving metformin. *Archives of Internal Medicine* 166: 1975–1079.

World Health Organization (WHO)/International Society for Hypertension (2003) Statement on the management of hypertension. *Journal of Hypertension* 21(11): 1983–1992.

Recommended reading

Buse J (2001) Insulin analogues. *Current Opinion in Endocrinology* 8(2): 95–100.

Campbell J, Anderson D, Holcombe J *et al.* (1993) Storage of insulin: a manufacturer's view. *Practical Diabetes* 10(6): 218–220.

Dunning T (2005) *Nursing Care of Older People with Diabetes.* Blackwell Publishing, Oxford.

Katz C (1991) How efficient is sliding scale insulin therapy? Problem with 'cookbook' approach in hospital patients. *Postgraduate Medicine* 5(5): 46–48.

Marks S (2000) Obesity management. *Current Therapeutics* 41: 6.

Independent medicine information

Australian Medicines Handbook (*www.amh.net.au*)
Australian Prescriber (*www.australianprescriber.com*)
National Prescribing Service (*www.nps.org.au*)
RADAR: updates on new medicines (*www.npsradar.org.au*)
The Cochrane Collaboration (*www.cochrane.org*)
Therapeutic Guidelines: Endocrinology (*www.tg.com.au*)

Chapter 6

Short-term complications

Key points

- Insulin should never be stopped in type 1 diabetes.
- People should be educated about and plan ahead for sick days and have a sick day kit ready.
- Hypoglycaemia is feared by people with diabetes and can compromise metabolic control and contribute to weight gain due to eating to manage the hypoglycaemia.
- Health professionals need to be aware of and sensitive about the psychological effects of hypoglycaemia, especially in type 1 diabetes and people with hypoglycaemic unawareness.

Introduction

Diabetes-related complications can occur in the short term and resolve, for example hypoglycaemia and hyperglycaemia-related events such as ketoacidosis (DKA), or as long-term complication such as cardiovascular disease. Short-term complications often result in considerable morbidity, can be frightening for individuals and their families, contribute to poor control, and contribute to falls risk and trauma and increase the likelihood of admission to hospital for older people.

The main short-term complications are:

- hypoglycaemia, which is the most significant complication associated with tight blood glucose control. In fact, hypoglycaemia is one of the barriers to achieving tight control (Diabetes Control and Complications Trial (DCCT) 1993);
- hyperglycaemia-related emergencies such as dehydration, DKA and hyperosmolar states;
- compromised immune system, which leads to delayed wound healing and infections such as urinary tract infections and respiratory diseases;

- acute changes in mental status, which affect self-care and decision-making in the short term and mean the individual may need assistance to manage and can be distressing in public situations and in the workplace.

Hypoglycaemia

Hypoglycaemia is usually defined as a blood glucose level < 3.0 mmol/L and is usually associated with symptoms related to the effects of the catecholamine hormones and sympathetic nervous system activity (Dunning 2003; Jenkins and O'Neal 2007). However, the blood glucose level at which symptoms occur varies among individuals and is affected by the rate at which the blood glucose falls, recent control, and the presence of autonomic neuropathy. Experts refer to Whipple's triad:

(1) the presence of low blood glucose;
(2) the presence of symptoms; and
(3) symptoms resolve when the blood glucose returns to the normal range.

Symptoms include sweating, anxiety, trembling, palpitations, slurred speech, uncoordinated movements, and behaviour changes which progresses to seizures and coma if glucose is not administered.

Nocturnal hypoglycaemia is often not recognised and the individual often does not wake and may not recall the episode afterwards. Indicators of nocturnal hypoglycaemia include restlessness, sweating, sleep disturbances such as vivid dreams, nightmares, a hung over sensation the following morning, depression, fatigue, and difficulty concentrating in the daytime. Common causes of nocturnal hypoglycaemia include exercise the preceding day, alcohol, and sometimes sexual activity.

Preventing hypoglycaemia is one of the most significant issues in diabetes self-management. It is sometimes difficult to achieve a balance between preventing hypoglycaemia and controlling hyperglycaemia to achieve HbA_{1c} targets and maintain quality of life, health and well-being. Hypoglycaemia occurred much more frequently in the intensive treatment group in the DCCT than in the control group: 61.2 episodes per 100 person years compared with 18.7. Health professionals need to understand the causes and psychological impact of hypoglycaemia to help the individual develop preventive strategies and treatment protocols.

Causes of hypoglycaemia

It is sometimes very difficult to identify a specific single cause. Hypoglycaemia can occur in people with diabetes treated with insulin, sulphonylureas, thiazolidinediones (TZDs) or glitinides. It is rare in people treated with metformin, but can occur. Hypoglycaemia can occur as a consequence of:

- very tight glycaemic control;
- missing or delaying meals;
- not eating sufficient carbohydrate;
- administering too much insulin or oral hypoglycaemic agent, which is common and usually accidental. In fact insulin is associated with the top 10 medicine-related errors people with diabetes and health professionals make (Hahn 2007);
- consuming alcohol on an empty stomach;
- reducing oral corticosteroid doses without reducing insulin or glucose-lowering medicines (see Chapter 5);
- suddenly losing weight without reducing insulin or oral medicine doses;
- medicine interactions including with some complementary glucose-lowering herbal medicines (see Chapter 11) and medicines such as non-cardiac selective beta blockers;
- prolonged or strenuous exercise, where it often occurs 6–8 hours after the exercise;
- frequent, prolonged hypoglycaemia;
- gastrointestinal disease such as coeliac disease and delayed gastric emptying due to autonomic neuropathy; and
- thyroid disease.

In older people sudden verbal or physical aggression may indicate hypoglycaemia. Some oral hypoglycaemic agents are contraindicated in older people with diabetes and concomitant renal or cardiovascular disease. For example, glibenclamide can cause prolonged hypoglycaemia because of its prolonged half-life, especially if renal disease is present. The hypoglycaemia presentation can be atypical and be mistaken for stroke, erratic behaviour, and wandering, which delay appropriate management and significantly affect quality of life.

Management consists of consuming oral glucose in mild episodes where the person is conscious, followed by more substantial carbohydrate to prevent the blood glucose from falling again. In severe episodes when the conscious state is affected, the airway must be cleared and maintained and IM glucagon or IV dextrose administered followed by oral carbohydrate once the person recovers enough to eat. The blood glucose should be checked regularly for 4–6 hours to ensure the hypo does not recur. In all cases strategies should be implemented to prevent further episodes. However, given the current focus on stringent blood glucose control some hypoglycaemia is unavoidable.

Hypoglycaemic unawareness

People with type 1 diabetes are prone to hypoglycaemic unawareness with long duration of diabetes. With increasing duration of type 1 diabetes the counter-regulatory response to hypoglycaemia diminishes (Cryer *et al.* 2003). All three counter-regulatory hormones are affected: glucagon release is impaired soon after diagnosis and progressively diminishes after 25 years' duration after which adrenalin becomes the main stress hormone released during hypoglycaemia. However, adrenalin release also diminishes over time. Adrenalin is responsible for most of the early signs of hypoglycaemia. In addition the neural response to hypoglycaemia gradually diminishes, so mild hypoglycaemia is not recognised or treated and progresses to severe hypoglycaemia and unconsciousness. Mild hypoglycaemia further impairs the counter-regulatory response especially if the hypoglycaemia is recurrent, which sets up a vicious cycle.

Hypoglycaemic unawareness is a risk factor for serious hypoglycaemia, cardiac arrhythmias, cognitive impairment and coma. Hypoglycaemic unawareness occurs in 25–33% of people with type 1 diabetes. As a consequence many people deliberately run their blood glucose high to avoid subsequent events. Management consists of:

- educating individuals and their families and carers to recognise situations likely to lead to hypos, and other cues to falling blood glucose;
- preventing episodes by avoiding alcohol on an empty stomach;
- reviewing insulin regimen (long-acting analogues reduce the risk of nocturnal hypoglycaemia); and
- diet review such as DAFNE.

The person should be counselled to wear a medical alert and use alarm devices such as Sleep Sentry. Companion animals, especially dogs, have been known to recognise hypoglycaemia and alert their owners or relatives. Hypos may mean the person is not able to drive for at least a year in some countries.

Continuous glucose monitoring system (CGMS) provides useful insight into blood glucose fluctuations in response to food, exercise, medications and other factors and identifies asymptomatic events. It can help appropriately tailor the management regimen. The monitor is usually worn for 72 hours and records the glucose every 5–10 minutes. The CGM sensor was not TGA approved in Australia at the time of writing.

Hyperglycaemia

Symptoms of hyperglycaemia – polyuria, polydipsia and lethargy – usually occur when blood glucose levels are > 15 mmol/L. Hyperglycaemia can be transient or occur over a longer time and can have significant long-term consequences. It may present as wandering, confusion and lethargy in older people. Hyperglycaemia is associated with increased morbidity and mortality in hospitalised patients and a range of medical and surgical conditions (American College of Endocrinology 2003). Associated morbid conditions include heart failure, wound and generalised infections, acute renal failure and delayed or non-recovery from vascular events, longer intubation times, longer length of stay and therefore increased costs.

It is important to determine whether the hyperglycaemia is the individual's usual blood glucose pattern (from HbA_{1c} and home monitoring record book) or occurred as a result of the hospital admission. Anxiety, reduced mobility, pain, especially angina, infection and some medications or treatments contribute to hyperglycaemia. An admission to hospital represents an opportunity to reassess diabetes management practices, knowledge, self-care and problem-solving ability including the sick day management plan, and diabetes complication and comorbidity status. Referral to a diabetes educator, dietitian or endocrinologist may be required.

Causes of hyperglycaemia

Causes of hyperglycaemia include:

- infection or acute illness, which is the most common cause;
- undiagnosed or newly diagnosed diabetes;
- inappropriate dietary intake;
- inappropriate or insufficient medication treatment;
- immobility;
- prolonged stress;
- corticosteroid and other diabetogenic medicines such as atypical antipsychotics (Koller and Doraiswamy 2002; Livingstone and Rampes 2004); and

- unrecognised insulin delivery system malfunction or changing to a different insulin delivery device especially where the individual's technique is not checked.

Hyperglycaemia can also occur when hospital staff do not check the person's technique or refer them for education, which increases the potential for repeat admissions and unnecessary investigations (Bhardwaj *et al.* 2006).

Hyperglycaemia management consists of:

- managing the acute episode and identifying and treating the underlying cause. This includes screening for an intercurrent illness, pain, or psychological stress. In hospital, intravenous insulin/glucose infusion is recommended (see Box 6.1);
- adjusting the diet if necessary;
- increasing exercise/activity; and
- reviewing and/or changing the medication regimen.

Box 6.1 Indications for continuous intravenous insulin infusion in inpatients with diabetes to manage hyperglycaemia

Maintaining the blood glucose at < 6 mmol/L reduces mortality and morbidity in critically ill patients. It is advisable that specific protocols be developed and agreed by relevant stakeholders (American Association of Clinical Endocrinologists 2003).

Medical conditions, including:

- any critical illness
- ketoacidosis
- hyperosmolar states
- lactic acidosis
- severe generalised infections and wound infections causing hyperglycaemia
- total parenteral nutrition
- prolonged fasting in people with or at risk of diabetes (insulin deficient states)
- myocardial infarction
- cerebrovascular events
- some high dose medicines such as glucocorticoids that induce hyperglycaemia

Surgical conditions, including:

- some investigative procedures
- perioperative period
- organ transplants

Labour and delivery in women with diabetes

Treating hyperglycaemia

Moderate hyperglycaemia (blood glucose approximately 10–15 mmol/L) accompanying acute illness or infection needs to be recognised and treated early to prevent ketoacidotic or hyperosmolar states. Hyperglycaemia with ketones or hyperosmolar states are more serious and require immediate medical management, which might involve increasing medicine doses or instituting insulin, or an insulin infusion, depending on the level of acidosis or dehydration and underlying cause. Blood glucose should be monitored at least 2- to 4-hourly depending on the severity of the event. Ketones should be monitored at the same time especially in type 1 diabetes. Note that the capillary blood glucose tests may be lower than the actual levels in the presence of high ketones. Blood ketones should be checked to guide management.

Preventing hyperglycaemia

Preventing hyperglycaemia is essential to preventing long-term complications. The person's ability to self-manage their medicines and optimal health professional prescribing are important aspects of management. The UKPDS demonstrated that progressive beta cell failure occurs in the majority of people with type 2 diabetes with increasing duration of diabetes, and insulin is required. Complications, especially renal failure, may necessitate a change to insulin. Commencing insulin therapy in people with type 2 diabetes can be challenging, but failure to prescribe insulin when OHA failure is evident increases the risk of short and long-term complications and reduces quality of life (see Chapter 8). Preventive general health measures are also important, such as influenza vaccine in at-risk individuals .

It should be noted that urine testing for glucose is inaccurate, especially in older people due to the raised renal threshold for glucose. A raised blood glucose level is often not detected in urine. Capillary and venous blood glucose testing and HbA_{1c} are the only accurate methods of determining the degree and duration of hyperglycaemia. People should be encouraged to develop a sick day management plan and to have a sick day kit prepared. Sometimes the best option may be to call the family or the doctor. Importantly insulin should not be stopped in type 1 diabetes.

Hyperglycaemic emergencies

Diabetic ketoacidosis

Diabetic ketoacidosis (DKA) usually occurs in people with type 1 diabetes, but DKA can occur in people with type 2 diabetes (Malone *et al.* 1992; Bagg *et al.* 1998; Newton and Raskin 2004). DKA occurs as a consequence of insulin deficiency and the production of large quantities of ketone bodies. Slim, older adults who are and have a history of weight loss are sometimes misdiagnosed as having type 2 diabetes and commenced on oral glucose-lowering medicines when they actually have latent autoimmune diabetes in adults (LADA) (see Chapter 2). These people often need insulin within weeks or months of diagnosis and can become acidotic if insulin is not commenced, especially if they become unwell. Table 6.1 shows the signs and symptoms of DKA and hyperosmolar states.

Hyperosmolar states

Hyperosmolar states most commonly occur in older people, often in previously undiagnosed people, in the presence of severe stress states such as infection, pneumonia, extensive burns, myocardial infarction,

Table 6.1 Comparison of the signs and symptoms of ketoacidosis and hyperosmolar states.

Ketoacidosis	Hyperosmolar states
Thirst	Polyuria
Polyuria	Glycosuria
Glycosuria	May not recognise thirst
Ketonuria	Dehydration
Fatigue	Extreme hyperglycaemia
Hyperglycaemia	Confusion
Nausea and vomiting	Elevated serum osmolality > 330 mOsmol/L
Abdominal pain	Coma (in late stages)
Muscle cramps	Biochemistry
Tachycardia	Elevated serum osmolality
Drowsiness	Elevated urea
Kussmaul's respirations (absent in late stages)	pH normal
Ketotic breath	
Biochemistry	
pH < 7.3 (significant ketosis)	

which may be silent, and reduced fluid intake in hot weather, which is frequently due to unrecognised thirst. Some medicines such as thiazide diuretics, corticosteroids, immunosuppressants, glucose dialysate fluids and parenteral nutrition can also precipitate hyperosmolar states (Braaten 1987).

Lactic acidosis

Lactic acidosis is less common than DKA and hyperosmolar states. Lactic acidosis can occur in acute illness where vasoconstriction, hypotension, liver cirrhosis and renal or liver impairment occur, and is an uncommon side effect of biguanides (Calabrese *et al.* 2002) when it does occur, it is usually in the presence of significant renal, hepatic or cardiac disease.

Management of all three states involves fluid, insulin and potassium replacement, preferably via an insulin infusion, and close monitoring of the metabolic status.

CASE DISCUSSION

Miss ME

Miss ME was referred to an endocrinologist and diabetes educator by her GP
Miss ME is a 28-year-old woman who has had type 1 diabetes since she was 10. She has good control on Mixtard 30/70 twice a day and her latest HbA_{1c} is 6.0%. Most of her home tests range between 4 and 6 mmol/L.

She exercises regularly and follows an appropriate diet. She reported frequent hypos but said she could cope with them. Her insulin dose was reduced and she was referred to the dietitian. She is very weight- and clothes-conscious.

In the past 2 months she has been admitted to the emergency department several times with severe hypoglycaemia including at night. She says her hypo symptoms are changing and she has trouble testing her BGs when her blood glucose is low.

She was changed to a basal bolus regime but the hypos continued, the latest causing convulsions.

Please advise what we can do next.

Dietitian

We have an experienced, possibly obsessive person here, so it is unlikely that she does not understand diabetes and only needs re-education. It is imperative that we stop the hypoglycaemia. Pre- and postprandial testing around meals could help determine the duration of action of her rapid-acting insulin and whether we need to reduce her basal insulin to stop nocturnal hypos.

I would initially check her eating pattern, carbohydrate intake and amount, duration, and timing of exercise and include a little supper until the nocturnal hypoglycaemia stops. She may not reduce her insulin enough on the days she does heavy exercise and experience delayed hypoglycaemia from the exercise. Hypoglycaemia can occur many hours after exercise. Usually basal bolus regimens and adjusting the insulin dose and carbohydrate on exercise days improves the situation.

Miss ME exercises regularly, which improves insulin sensitivity, so she is likely to need smaller doses of insulin. She may have been given inappropriate education regarding exercise and insulin in the past and need re-education about sport, diet, including carbohydrate intake such as the amount, type, GI effect, meal distribution during the day, when to eat, and insulin dose adjustment on high exercise days, as well as delayed hypoglycaemia.

I would consider referring her to a psychologist. She is weight- and clothes-conscious. She may have a disordered body image and may have an eating disorder, which needs to be explored by assessing her diet history, which may not be accurate initially. There is also a need to consider how she lives, with whom she lives and what she means when she says she 'copes' with hypos. She may be seeking attention.

Diabetes educator

Diabetes clinical nurse consultants see many young women such as Miss ME who need understanding and support. I would complete an education assessment and find out what she hopes to achieve. The assessment would include usual demographic details, living situation, work and lifestyle, diabetes and treatment status, blood glucose testing practices, activity levels, weight history, eating, alcohol consumption, and smoking status (see Figure 3.1). Asking about stress and using a Likert scale to assess how Miss ME copes with diabetes could be helpful. Other health history includes the number and frequency of hypoglycemia and ketoacidosis events, and medications. I would ask about over-the-counter treatments and complementary therapies because people may not volunteer such information. The assessment will determine mutual actions to be achieved from the consultation, plans for the next consultation, and what resources and referrals to other team members might be required (see Figure 3.1). Teaching checklists can save time and repetition.

Several consultations will enable a rapport to be developed and time to discuss Miss ME's interests such as the latest colours and fashions. Initiating a basal bolus regimen using a peakless long-acting insulin before bed does not seem to have prevented nocturnal hypoglycaemia. Miss ME may have been brought up by her parents to keep her diabetes under 'tight control' for fear of complications such as blindness and amputation and perhaps not being able to have a family. The benefits of psychological counselling should be discussed with her.

I would download her blood glucose test results from her meter, but would be prepared for few episodes of hypoglycaemia to be recorded. While she may carry her meter with her, the hypoglycaemic autonomic symptoms of sweating, trembling, anxiety and nausea and the fact that the hypos occur at night may mean she is not able to test her blood glucose until she recovers, which could be some hours later, when the blood glucose is high due to the counter-regulatory response or returned to normal.

Continuous glucose monitoring (CGM), involving a small device clipped to the belt connected to a small sensor electrode inserted under the skin, could provide useful information about her blood glucose pattern. The meter is worn continuously, usually 72 hours, and interstitial glucose is measured every 5 minutes. The insertion process only takes a few minutes but an initial 1-hour calibration period is required.

I would also discuss the possible benefits of an insulin pump. The pump is attached to an infusion line inserted under the skin. The basal rate delivers insulin continuously and several different rates can be programmed over the course of the day. Bolus doses are delivered by pressing a button to deliver a specific amount of insulin at each meal, taking into account carbohydrate intake, blood glucose level, and exercise. Correction boluses can be given when the blood glucose levels are too high and during illness.

There are several ways to work out the best formula for each person's pump and to deliver the appropriate insulin dose. Frequent blood glucose testing is needed initially to enable insulin and other adjustments to be made. The pump is disconnected for showers and the spa, some sports and sometimes during intimacy. Alarms alert the person to pump malfunctions such as the infusion tubing disconnecting from the pump or low batteries. Meticulous insertion technique is necessary and the cannula and tubing should be changed every 2–3 days. Insulin pumps can improve lifestyle by enabling greater flexibility. In addition, Miss ME may regain her ability to detect hypoglycaemia symptoms. I would refer her to a dietitian, especially if she chose to use a pump, and suggest a dose adjusted for normal eating (DAFNE) programme.

Diabetes educator 2

I agree with most of these suggestions, but two other issues are worth exploring: these include whether the hypoglycaemia is related to alcohol intake or sexual activity. Both are very sensitive issues and need to be discussed tactfully and in a non-judgemental way. She might also benefit from blood glucose awareness training (BGAT) (Cox *et al.* 2001). Islet cell transplantation could be considered if all the suggested options do not improve the situation.

Psychologist

It is likely that Miss ME is suffering from two inter-related challenges. First, she may have lost her sensitivity to hypoglycaemia (hypoglycaemia awareness), which is not uncommon among people with long-standing diabetes, especially those who have managed to maintain good control of their diabetes. This means that she may be having many mild hypoglycaemic episodes without being aware of them, which might explain the good HbA_{1c} despite the episodes of DKA. The second challenge is her anxiety over having hypoglycaemia, and subsequent running of high blood glucose values. Combined, these two challenges can provide an interacting spiral that drive the person down emotionally and drive the blood glucose levels high.

One traditional way to address hypoglycaemia unawareness is to support individuals running their blood glucose levels high for an extended period of time, until they regain their sensitivity to mild hypoglycaemia. However, if someone has microvascular complications, this period of elevated blood glucose levels may exacerbate the progression of complications. An alternative approach would be to help people learn to regain their awareness through a focused self-management programme. Blood glucose awareness training (BGAT) (Cox *et al.* 2001) and its derivatives such as hypoglycaemia awareness training (HAT) (Kinsley *et al.* 1999) have demonstrated remarkable efficacy in helping people regain their hypo awareness. Some of the studies have indicated that these programmes do more than reskill the individual to identify his/her hypo symptoms more readily, and may facilitate the recovery of neuroendocrine responses to low blood glucose levels (Kinsley *et al.* 1999).

Running programmes such as these with demonstrable efficacy may be difficult to implement in practice – due to lack of training, difficulty accessing the programme and insufficient resources. In addition, people may not want to take part in such intensive programmes.

Key aspects of the programme could be evaluated in individual consultations. Although no trials have been published using this approach, it may be of real value to combine the body scan and error grid analysis with individual patients. Patients scan their body for any symptoms they notice at that time. Based on this and their knowledge of their insulin, diet and activity over the day, they then estimate their blood glucose values. If they do this repeatedly, they can learn to identify those symptoms consistently related to high blood glucose values and those related to low glucose values This, in theory, along with self-management education around how to adjust insulin levels proactively for food and activity levels, could have a substantial impact on Miss ME's anxiety and diabetes glucose regulation.

CASE DISCUSSION

> **Mr BR**
>
> ***Mr BR's parents telephoned the diabetes educator for advice following a severe hypoglycaemic episode***
> Mr BR is an 18-year-old male. His parents found him comatose when they tried to wake him for school. He had attended a school leavers' party with his friends the night before and the friends knew he had had quite a bit of alcohol and danced most of the evening but were not sure whether he had eaten anything.
> The parents could not rouse him, even by putting honey in his mouth, so they drove him to the ER.
> His blood glucose was 1.4 mmol/L and he responded to IM glucagon.

Diabetes educator

Mr BR probably realises the seriousness of this experience but may not realise the effect of alcohol and exercise on his blood glucose levels. I would explore these issues with him and suggest ways to manage social events in the future. These include eating sufficient carbohydrate during the evening or having high-calorie soft drinks and adjusting his insulin levels. He should realise other dangers in such situations such as possible accidents, being mugged and should be aware of the dangers of hypoglycaemia, alcohol and driving. The episode may need to be reported to the road traffic authority, which would mean he could not drive until his blood glucose was stable again. Wearing some form of identification that he has diabetes is advisable. I would tactfully ask about drug use.

It is important that he has a trusted friend who can help him in such emergencies and knows how to manage Mr BR should he become unconscious and the emergency telephone number to call.

The friend and parents may benefit from learning how to use glucagon. He may benefit from a consultation with a dietitian and/or BGAT education and his parents may need support.

CASE DISCUSSION

Mrs PJ

Mrs PJ was referred to the diabetes centre by a physician in the infectious diseases department of a large metropolitan hospital
Mrs PJ is an 80-year-old woman who has had type 1 diabetes for 54 years. She lives with her son, who is single. Her son draws up her insulin in a syringe and Mrs PJ administers it herself.

Mrs PJ had a hypo while she was attending the infectious diseases clinic and was referred to you for education about hypoglycaemia.

As you discuss the hypo episode with her, you discover she has frequent hypoglycaemic episodes and no longer recognises hypoglycaemic symptoms.

She tells you her blood glucose levels change rapidly, which she finds frustrating.

She has osteomyelitis of the left heel, which is why she is attending the infectious diseases clinic.

You note in her medical record that she has chronic renal impairment (creatinine 295, normal 50–100).

She has had a recent presentation to the emergency department with unstable angina refractory to anginine and has a past history of non-ST elevation myocardial infarction (NSTEMI).

The medical notes indicate she was 'Given isolated, extra doses of actrapid according to the blood glucose' while in emergency.

Her son reports he gives an extra dose of Actrapid whenever Mrs PJ's blood glucose is > 12 mmol/L.

Current medications

Aspirin	100 mg/day
Atorvastatin	40 mg nocte
Caltrate	1 tablet/day
Calcitriol	1 tablet mane
Omeprazole	20 mg/day
Diltiazem	60 mg BD
Paracetamol	QID (strict)
Ciprofloxacin	500 mg BD
Augmentin	BD
Furosemide	200 mg mane, 160 mg midday, 160 mg nocte
Spironolactone	12.5 mg/day

Protaphane	24 units mane
Actrapid	3–5 units mane but the son gives extra Actrapid at home when the blood glucose goes above 10 mmol/L
Glyceryl trinitrate patch	10 mg
Metoprolol	100 mg mane

Diabetes educator

I would ascertain her latest HbA_{1c}, or order one if there was no recent result: 54 years of type 1 diabetes means 54 years of hypoglycaemia. However, with recent new insulins now available, this scenario can be changed. Neither Actrapid nor Protaphane are the insulins of choice. Both are extremely variable with respect to when their actions start, when they peak and how long they last. Actrapid peaks 4 hours after administration, which for most people means just before lunch. People with diabetes who are prescribed Actrapid must eat a snack within 3 hours of administering this insulin and can rarely afford to prolong the time they have their lunch or evening meal. When administering Actrapid with the evening meal, a significant supper is also required to prevent hypoglycaemia.

Protaphane generally starts to work within 2 hours of administration and can peak in its action anywhere from 4–12 hours. This means that later in the afternoon, Mrs PJ could in fact be having her lunchtime Actrapid and her breakfast Protaphane peaking at the same time, creating a profound hypoglycaemic effect. It is also important to note that the entire regimen appears quite unusual. People with type 1 diabetes often take Protaphane at bedtime, rather than in the morning. At present Mrs PJ has no overnight insulin and could be starting each day with raised blood glucose levels. This could also be affecting her sleeping patterns if overnight hyperglycaemia and subsequent polyuria is causing her to use the toilet frequently overnight. Waking with raised blood glucose levels may in turn be giving a false impression of her actual glycaemic control and insulin requirements and therefore means that much larger doses of insulin are administered in the morning to 'try to catch up' with morning hyperglycaemia.

There are also several other considerations. How many extra doses of Actrapid is Mrs PJ giving herself? When is she monitoring her blood glucose levels and does this coincide with the peak action of her insulin? For example, if following breakfast Actrapid, Mrs PJ tests her blood glucose levels and they are above 12 mmol/L, does she administer herself more insulin? This is potentially very dangerous and also helps to explain why sliding scales of Actrapid will never achieve good and safe glycaemic control. The peak action time of Actrapid is usually 4 hours after administration; taking a blood glucose level only 2 hours after means that the peak action of Actrapid has not yet occurred. Giving extra Actrapid at this time markedly increases the risk of hypoglycaemia occurring.

Another consideration is that she is being treated for osteomyelitis. Infection usually causes a marked rise in blood glucose levels. More insulin is often required to address infection-induced hyperglycaemia. Mrs PJ's osteomyelitis may now be resolving and therefore her insulin requirements will need to be reduced. It would also be useful to identify whether other infections were present, for example a urinary tract infection where symptoms of polyuria may be masked due to hyperglycaemia and diuretic therapy and thrush resulting from current antibiotic treatment.

There is no mention of her level of cognition. Performing a Mini-Mental State Examination (MMSE) is imperative to determine the level of understanding she has and the degree of insight into her condition. Vascular dementia is a long-term complication of diabetes and she already exhibits other vascular complications: NSTEMI and chronic renal failure.

I would change Mrs PJ to a basal analog and bolus analog. Lantus at breakfast should provide 24 hours coverage as the basal insulin and markedly reduce any nocturnal hypoglycaemia. Daily glargine in older people is associated with fewer hypoglycaemic episodes and improvements in blood glucose control (Janka *et al.* 2005). NovoRapid or Humalog insulin with each meal can provide more timely coverage of postprandial excursions in blood glucose control, reduce the need to snack between meals and provide more flexibility with meal times.

A short hospital admission may be useful to carefully monitor insulin regimen changes. Self-insulin administration could be observed, sites of injections could be examined for hypertrophy and hypoglycaemic management in terms of treatment and prevention could be revised. Such a short admission could also bring a much-needed team approach:

- an endocrinologist to review insulin regimens;
- the diabetes educator to review knowledge and self-management skills;
- the dietitian to maximise nutritional intake for an older woman with chronic renal failure;
- the podiatrist to ensure modified footwear can be fitted to assist with wound healing and minimise wound breakdown; and

- a social worker to review Mrs PJ's home situation and identify any services she may need such as meals on wheels.

Osteomyelitis is a very difficult and challenging infection to treat and a course of intravenous antibiotics may prove a more useful intervention.

Time and resources must also be devoted to Mrs PJ's son to determine his level of understanding pertaining to his mother's diabetes and management. It would appear that he might have been following the emergency department intervention strategy of a sliding scale regimen. It is also important to identify whether anyone actually instructed him to use a sliding scale when his mother was discharged. This scenario is unfortunately common – medical and nursing staff do not always fully understand diabetes and its management and provide instructions that can then create the type of scenario we are now confronted with.

Her other medications need to be reviewed as follows:

- Atorvastatin needs to be monitored carefully in an 80-year-old with chronic renal failure. Both renal function and creatine kinase (CK) need to be measured regularly. There may be now little benefit to remain on this medication, or it may need to be reduced to a lower dose.
- Caltrate should be ceased as it is a contraindication when prescribed calcitriol. This is even more relevant in a frail older woman with chronic renal failure.
- Frusemide is ordered at night and I would question how an older woman is expected to sleep if she must get up to void frequently.
- Spironolactone may require to be reconsidered with respect to a frail older woman with poorly controlled type 1 diabetes due to a high risk of hyperkalaemia, respiratory or metabolic acidosis.
- Metoprolol may have a role in masking the symptoms of hypoglycaemia.

In conclusion, the management of older people with diabetes should be a team effort (Tattersall 1997).

Diabetes educator 2

I agree with this comprehensive assessment. Managing diabetes in older people is a complex and changing undertaking. Mrs PJ is 80; management needs to consider her life expectancy and prioritise her health risks and preferences. She may prefer to maintain her independence, which may be a key aspect of quality of life for her. The MMSE may or may not be helpful, depending on the conditions under which it is undertaken. If it occurs under 'ideal' conditions when her blood glucose is in the optimal range, for example after she was stabilised in hospital, she may perform well and be judged capable of self-care. However, if it was performed under 'usual' conditions such as at home a different result may be obtained. Serial MMSE tests may be more useful than a single test. It would also be important to undertake other activities of daily living (ADL) tests and these should also be performed at regular intervals. Mrs PJ's and her son's knowledge of diabetes and its management and insulin technique may need to be checked.

Her nutritional status needs to be considered and she may benefit from supplements to improve her wound healing capacity and overall health. If possible, the mental status of both Mrs PJ and her son should be assessed. Managing diabetes is a considerable burden and one or both may be suffering from depression. The focus is currently on her foot with the cellulitic heel. It is essential that both feet are monitored: it is not uncommon for the non-damaged foot to be neglected.

Podiatrist

Osteomyelitis of the heel has a poor prognosis. Mrs PJ's advanced age and the presence of renal disease suggest she has peripheral vascular disease, which will impair healing and reduce the effectiveness of systemic antibiotics. If not already undertaken, a thorough assessment should include palpating her pedal pulses. If they are weak or absent, an ankle brachial index followed by a duplex scan (if her arteries are calcified) will provide more information about her vascular status. If these tests indicate that Mrs PJ has peripheral arterial disease, she should be reviewed by a vascular specialist to determine whether revascularisation is possible to improve her blood supply and her healing potential.

While the infectious disease department is monitoring her antibiotic therapy, foot disease usually requires a multidisciplinary approach including debridement, wound care and pressure offloading. The degree of debridement required depends on the blood supply and extent of the necrosis. It may be performed by a podiatrist with expertise managing diabetic foot pathology or in an operating theatre by a vascular or orthopaedic surgeon if extensive debridement is indicated.

Wound care should include non-occlusive dressings changed every three days to control exudate, prevent maceration of the wound margin and maintain a slightly moist environment. However, if she has very poor circulation, non-adherent dry dressings are preferred. Pressure on the wound should be alleviated using in-bed appliances such as a foam tunnel to keep her heel off the bed. When walking, a specially padded healing shoe or a shoe with the heel cut away to reduce pressure on the heel is essential. Careful monitoring of the size, depth and appearance of the wound and underlying bony changes using X-rays is important. Surgical resection of the bone may be required if the osteomyelitis does not respond to antibiotics and the pressure and wound management strategies outlined.

CASE DISCUSSION

> *Telephone question to the diabetes educator from an ER nurse*
> I work in the ER and we heard about blood ketone testing at a recent inservice. Should we do that instead of testing urine?

Diabetes educator

Yes. Blood ketone testing in the ER is a useful, fast, and accurate way of detecting ketoacidosis (Naunheim *et al.* 2006). Blood ketone testing detects beta-hydroxybuterate (BOH), the most significant and abundant ketoacid, which is not detected via urine ketone test strips. The manufacturer suggests that ketones > 1.5 mmol/L indicate ketoacidosis. The ability to recognise ketoacidosis early may enable patients to be triaged faster, reduce waiting times in ER, and ensure treatment is instituted early. Increasingly people with type 1 diabetes are being taught to monitor blood ketones during illness.

References

American College of Endocrinology (2003) Proceedings of Consensus Development Conference on Inpatient Diabetes and Metabolic Control (www.aace.com).

Bagg W, Sathu A, Streat S *et al.* (1998) Diabetic ketoacidosis in adults at Auckland Hospital, 1988–1996. *Australian and New Zealand Journal of Medicine* 28(5): 604–608.

Bhardwaj V, Metcalfe N, Innes E *et al.* (2006) Recurrent diabetic ketoacidosis after changing pen devices for insulin injection. *British Medical Journal* 332: 1259–1260.

Braaten J (1987) Hyperosmolar non-ketonic diabetic coma: diagnosis and management. *Geriatrics* 42: 83–92.

Calabrese AT, Coley KC, DaPos S *et al.* (2002) Evaluation of prescribing practices: risk of lactic acidosis with metformin therapy. *Archives of Internal Medicine* 162: 434–437.

Cox D, Gonder-Frederick L, Polonsky W *et al.* (2001) Blood glucose awareness training (BGAT-2): long-term benefits. *Diabetes Care* 24(4): 637–642.

Cryer P, Davis S, Shamoon H (2003) Hypoglycaemia in diabetes. *Diabetes Care* 26: 1902–1912.

Diabetes Control and Complications Trial (DCCT) Research Group (1993) Epidemiology of severe hypoglycaemia in the diabetes control and complications trial. *American Journal of Medicine* 90: 450–459.

Dunning T (2003) *Care of People with Diabetes. A Manual of Nursing Practice.* Blackwell Publishing, Oxford.

Hahn K (2007) *The 'Top 10' Drug Errors and How to Prevent Them.* Proceedings of the American Pharmacists Association Annual Meeting, Atlanta, March.

Janka H, Plewe G, Busch K (2007) Combination of oral antidiabetic agents with basal insulin versus premixed insulin alone in elderly patients with type 2 diabetes. *Journal of the American Geriatrics Society* 55(2): 182–188.

Jenkins A, O'Neal D (2007) Hypoglycaemic unawareness. *Diabetes Management Journal* 18: 22.

Kinsley B, Weinger K, Baja M *et al.* (1999) Blood glucose awareness training and epinephrine responses to hypoglycaemia during intensive treatment in type 1 diabetes. *Diabetes Care* 22(7): 1022–1028.

Koller E, Doraiswamy P (2002) Olanzapine-associated diabetes mellitus. *Pharmacotherapy* 22(7): 841–852.

Livingstone C, Rampes H (2004) Atypical antipsychotic drugs and diabetes. *Practical Diabetes International* 20 (9): 237–331.

Malone M, Gennis V, Goodwin J (1992) Characteristics of diabetic ketoacidosis in older versus younger adults. *Journal of the American Geriatrics Society* 40: 1100–1104.

Naunheim R, Jang TJ, Banet G *et al.* (2006) Point-of-care test identifies diabetic ketoacidosis at triage. *Academic Emergency Medicine* 13: 683–685.

Newton C, Raskin P (2004) Diabetic ketoacidosis in type 1 and type 2 diabetes mellitus. Clinical and biochemical differences. *Archives of Internal Medicine* 164: 1925–1931.

Sinclair AJ, Finucane P (2001) *Diabetes in Old Age.* John Wiley and Sons, Chichester.

Tattersall R (1997) Improving treatment outcomes in the elderly. *Reducing the Burden of Diabetes* 11: 9–11.

Recommended reading

Australian Diabetes Educators Association (ADEA) (2006) *Guidelines for Sick Day Management for People with Diabetes*. ADEA, Canberra.

Dunning T (2003) *Care of People with Diabetes. A Manual of Nursing Practice*. Blackwell Publishing, Oxford.

Dunning T (2005) *Nursing Care of Older People with Diabetes*. Blackwell Publishing, Oxford.

Kitabachi A, Fisher J Murphy M *et al.* (1994) Diabetic ketoacidosis and the hyperglycaemic hyperosmolar nonketotic state. In Kahn L, Weir G (eds) *Joslin's Diabetes Mellitus*. Lea and Febiger, Philadelphia, pp 738–770.

Van Staa T, Abenhaim L, Monette J (1997) Risk factors for hypoglycaemia in users of sulphonylureas. Rates of hypoglycaemia in users of sulphonylureas. *Journal of Clinical Epidemiology* 50: 735–741.

Chapter 7

Long-term complications

Key points

- Good metabolic control reduces the risk of long-term complications.
- A prospective regular structured complication assessment programme is essential to improving outcomes. It should encompass psychological, spiritual, and social factors, and a comprehensive medication review.
- An holistic approach to managing complications is necessary.
- Complications may be 'silent'.
- Achieving 'good control' is hard work and is very difficult to sustain especially when complications are present.

Introduction

Prolonged hyperglycaemia results in a range of pathological, metabolic and mechanical changes that contribute to the development of diabetes complications. Diabetes complications cause a great deal of morbidity, including psychological stress and can reduce quality of life and life expectancy. Increasing age increases the risk and progression of micro and macrovascular complications and older people diagnosed with diabetes have more morbidity and lower life expectancy than non-diabetics of the same age (Bethel *et al.* 2007).

Causal mechanisms for long-term complications have been identified and are shown in Table 7.1. The presence of diabetes complications significantly increases the per-patient cost of managing diabetes (Bate and Jerums 2003). A multidisciplinary, multimodal approach is necessary, but achieving stringent blood pressure, blood glucose, and lipid targets is difficult to achieve and sustain.

Three broad levels of susceptibility have been described:

(1) five percent of people with diabetes develop complications even after relatively brief, mild hyperglycaemia;
(2) twenty percent tolerate prolonged hyperglycaemia; and

Table 7.1 Significant actual (proven) risk factors that could contribute to the development of the long-term complications of diabetes. Many of the potential risk factors are difficult to measure in routine clinical practice.

Factors that actually represent significant risk	Possible contributing factors
High LDL cholesterol	Oxidative stress and the generation of reactive oxygen species, which increases the formation of advanced glycated end products (AGE)
High triglycerides	Increased tissue glycosylation, which also contributes to AGE
Low HDL cholesterol	Inflammatory disease, which promotes the formation of proinflammatory cytokines, chemokines, and adhesion molecules
Elevated blood pressure	Impaired vasodilation and calcification of blood vessels
Smoking	Adhesion molecules
Persistent hyperglycaemia, which causes a cascade of metabolic disturbances	Plasminogen activator inhibitor-1 (PAI-1)
Insulin resistance and hyperinsulinaemia	Elevated vasoconstrictor levels such as E-selection
Genetic predisposition	

(3) seventy-five percent have moderate degrees of susceptibility, and intensive blood glucose, lipid, and blood pressure control may prevent or delay the onset of complications in this group (Raskin and Rosenstock 1992).

The Diabetes Control and Complications Trial (DCCT) (1993) in type 1 diabetes and the United Kingdom Prospective Diabetes Study (UKPDS) (1998) demonstrated that controlling the underlying metabolic abnormalities ($HbA_{1c} < 7\%$) reduced complications and improved long-term outcomes. In the DCCT, microangiopathy was reduced by 39%, neuropathy by 60%, risk of developing retinopathy by 76% and retinopathy progression by 54%. However, only a minority, 37%, actually sustained $HbA_{1c} < 7\%$. The UKPDS demonstrated a reduction in microvascular complications: retinopathy by 25%, erectile dysfunction by 20% and macrovascular disease by 40% by controlling hyperglycaemia and significantly, by lowering blood pressure.

The main long-term complications of diabetes are:

• macrovascular disease such as stroke and cardiac disease;

- microvascular disease such as nephropathy and retinopathy, which often coexist especially in type 1 diabetes; and
- neuropathy:
  - *peripheral*, leading to foot pathology
  - *autonomic*, which causes gastroparesis, unrecognised hypoglycaemia, erectile dysfunction (ED), silent myocardial infarct (MI), and silent urinary tract infection (UTI).

Other less commonly discussed but equally important complications are dental disease, cataracts, musculoskeletal conditions, and psychological distress, all of which impact on self-care and affect the individual's ability to achieve the recommended management targets and sustain them in the long term.

Priorities include:

- prevention through early identification of people at risk using regular, structured screening programmes;
- early treatment of underlying pathology;
- improving blood glucose and lipids;
- managing hypertension;
- diabetes education;
- nutritional assessment;
- regular medication reviews; and
- psychosocial evaluation.

As function is compromised, rehabilitation programmes and assistance with self-care and activities of daily living (ADL) may be needed.

Cardiovascular disease

The CADILLAC (Controlled Abciximab and Device Investigation to Lower Late Angioplasty Complications) trial showed that cardiovascular disease particularly heart failure and myocardial infarction (MI) frequently result in hospital admissions and death in people with diabetes (Stuckey *et al.* 2005). The presence of cardiovascular disease may affect self-care ability, exercise capacity, increase the risk of comorbidities such as falls in older people, and influences medication choices and doses. People with diabetes have more extensive and severe atherosclerosis in their coronary and cerebral blood vessels than non-diabetics. In addition, autonomic neuropathy can give rise to atypical presentations of cardiovascular disease (silent MI) and lead to delayed treatment and sudden death. Over 50% of type 2 deaths result from cardiovascular disease and people with diabetes often die before they reach hospital.

Table 7.2 outlines risk factors for cardiovascular disease. There is a spectrum of risk that encompasses medical and lifestyle factors, family history of cardiovascular disease, and genetic predisposition, for example familial hyperlipidaemia. Significantly, the lifetime risk of death for women with diabetes is the same as for men. Premenopausal women and women on hormone replacement (oestrogen and selective estrogen receptor modulators, SERMs) have the same risk as men. Recently the American Heart Association revised its guidelines for preventing cardiovascular disease in women. The revised guidelines focus on women's lifetime risk of heart disease because the lifetime risk of dying from heart disease is nearly 1:3 (Mosca 2007).

The guidelines include a recommendation to consider low-dose aspirin in women over 65 years regardless of their cardiovascular status and increasing the upper dose for women at high risk of cardiovascular disease to 325 mg/day (Mosca 2007). Aspirin may not be necessary for healthy women < 65 years. The guidelines also underscored the importance of:

- adopting a healthy lifestyle for women of all ages (diet and regular activity) (see Chapter 4);
- managing blood pressure;
- weight control;
- reducing sodium and alcohol intake;
- consuming a diet rich in fruit and vegetables, low in saturated fat (7%), including omega-3 oils at least twice per week and eicosapentaenoic acid (EPA) supplements 850–1000 mg. Antioxidant supplements were not recommended;
- controlling fasting plasma glucose; and
- being cautious about using hormone replacement therapy.

MI is 'silent' in 32% of people with diabetes. 'Silent infarct' is a term used to describe the vague symptoms people with diabetes can experience during an MI. The classical cardiac pain across the chest, down the arm, and into the jaw may not be present in people with diabetes. They often mistake the discomfort for indigestion and delay seeking help (Dunning and Martin 1998). The atypical nature of the chest pain makes it difficult for people to accept that they had a heart attack and they may not understand why they are being asked to modify risk factors. MI in older people may present as heart failure, cardiogenic shock, congestive cardiac failure (CCF), diabetic ketoacidosis, hyperosmolar coma or hypoglycaemia. Early cardiac investigations such as ECGs, angiograms, and stress tests are indicated and stents and coronary artery bypass grafts (CABGs) may be required.

Table 7.2 Risk factors for cardiovascular disease. People with long duration of diabetes and two to three risk factors present have the same risk as a non-diabetic person with one risk factor.

Risk factor	Effects
Hypertension	Thickened, less elastic blood vessels
	Increased strain on the heart
Left ventricular hypertrophy and calcification of the cardiac arteries, which is associated with duration of diabetes and the albumin creatinine ratio. Smoking is associated with the extent of calcification but not body mass index	Contributes to hypertension
Smoking	Contributes to hypertension
	Increased risk of cardiac disease, especially in women
	Increased risk of cancer
	Constricts blood vessels
Hyperlipidaemia	Significant positive predictor of cardiovascular disease
Dyslipidaemia	
Hyperglycaemia	
Coagulopathies	Plaque formation
	Emboli
Family history of cardiovascular disease	Increased risk of cardiovascular disease
Hyperglycaemia	Increased platelet aggregation
	Multiple effects on tissues and organs
Psychosocial factors	Some psychosocial factors are associated with increased cardiovascular risk including:
	– depression – social isolation – lack of support
	and may influence other risk factors such as smoking, overeating and inactivity
Obesity and inactivity	Cardiovascular disease
	Reduced exercise tolerance
Diabetes	Presence of diabetes eliminates female protection
Older age	

In addition, congestive heart failure occurs in 10–30% of people with diabetes and the prognosis is worse than in non-diabetics. Some medications such as thiazolidinediones (TZDs) may be contra-indicated, while diuretics, angiotensin-converting enzyme (ACE-I), reducing alcohol, and smoking are essential. Cardiomyopathy also occurs as a result of many cardiac events over time and other causes. Symptoms include tiredness, which can be mistaken for a number of unrelated conditions or exercise intolerance. Cardiomyopathy can occur early in diabetes and is not necessarily related to the presence of other complications, diabetes duration, or glycaemic control. A number of factors contribute to diastolic and systolic blood pressure abnormalities and abnormalities in heart muscle fibres that affect heart muscle contractility and relaxation and leads to stiffened ventricles. Factors contributing to cardiomyopathy include alcohol, negative inotropic medicines, thyroid disease, and haemochromatosis.

Management of cardiac disease is specific to the underlying abnormality(ies) but general management includes:

- controlling hypertension to reduce the risk of cardiac events and stroke (UK Prospective Diabetic Study (UKPDS) 1998);
- controlling blood glucose and lipids. Dyslipidaemia promotes lesion formation in coronary vessels. Statins contribute to secondary prevention and reduce cardiovascular risk including after CAGs (Goldberg *et al.* 1998; Hoogwerf *et al.* 1998; Long-term Intervention with Pravastatin in Ischaemic Heart Disease (LIPID) Study 1998);
- eating a low-fat, high-fibre diet;
- exercising within individual capacity. Exercise capacity is limited by the degree of cardiovascular disease and people should have a thorough assessment before embarking on an exercise programme (Van de Veire *et al.* 2006);
- quitting smoking – nicotine replacement therapy may help;
- drinking alcohol in moderation;
- medications such as beta blockers, ACE-I, diuretics, and vasodilators;
- education about reducing risks and recognising silent MI and the importance of seeking medical advice early;
- in the acute stages of an MI, an IV insulin/glucose infusion, frequent monitoring, and surgical interventions may be necessary. Subsequent subcutaneous insulin for about 3 months is associated with improved outcomes (Malmberg *et al.* 1999).

A significant proportion of people do not take their cardiovascular medicines in the long term, even though prescriptions for lipid-lowering agents, antihypertensive agents and OHAs have increased in accordance with best practice (Australian Institute of Health and Welfare (AIHW) 2007). This finding suggests that medicine reviews should be part of the long-term complication screening protocols.

Cerebrovascular disease

Stroke can be caused and preceded by hypertension. Almost every person who presents with a stroke has a history of hypertension. In older people stroke is a major cause of morbidity and mortality. Many older people fear having a stroke and consider it almost worse than dying from a stroke. Transient ischaemic attacks (TIAs) occur when the blood supply to a part of the brain is temporarily interrupted but does not cause permanent damage and recovery usually occurs within 24 hours. Frequent TIAs may indicate impending stroke. Small repeated strokes sometimes lead to progressive brain damage and multi-infarct dementia, which may present as:

- gradual memory loss
- diminished intellectual capacity
- loss of motor function
- incontinence.

Preventive management is essentially the same as for cardiovascular disease.

Nephropathy

Diabetic nephropathy is a significant diabetes microvascular complication and is the second most common cause of end-stage renal disease in Australia, New Zealand and the UK (ANZDATA 2000; Department of Health 2001). Microalbuminuria, an early marker of renal function decline, occurs in approximately 20% of people with diabetes: 40% eventually develop nephropathy. Aboriginal and Torres Strait Island peoples and Afro-Caribbeans are at increased risk of renal disease. There is a strong link between renal disease and retinopathy and cardiovascular disease.

Diabetic nephropathy is a chronic progressive disease usually divided into five stages:

(1) increased glomerular filtration rate (GFR);
(2) glomerular lesions and thickened basement membrane;
(3) incipient nephropathy where microalbuminuria is present and the albumin excretion rate (AER) is between 30 and 300 mg/day.

Microalbuminuria is associated with cardiovascular morbidity and mortality in type 2 diabetes (de Zeeuw *et al.* 2004);

(4) clinical nephropathy where proteinuria is overt and exceeds 500 mg/day and the GFR < 15 ml/minute; and

(5) end-stage renal disease (ESRD). When the GFR is < 10 ml/minute, dialysis is required.

Clinical renal disease is present in one-third of people with type 2 diabetes 10–20 years after the onset of diabetes and between 25 and 40% of type 1 after 25 years. Significant predictors of microalbuminuria include high AER, male gender, high arterial blood pressure, elevated HbA_{1c}, and short stature (Microalbuminuria Collaborative Study Group 1999). Recent studies suggest the rate of decline can be slowed and survival improved by identifying and treating micro and macrovascular disease (Hovind 2005). Measures of renal function include 12- and 24-hour and spot urine collections to measure microalbumin, creatinine, albumin/creatinine ratio, glomerular filtration rate (GFR) and e-GFR, which should be undertaken regularly.

Management is multifactorial. Prevention is paramount by controlling blood glucose, blood pressure and lipids, eating a healthy diet and reducing sodium intake. Secondary prevention includes antihypertensive agents such as ACE-I and/or angiotensin receptor blockers, for example irbesartan (Parving *et al.* 2001) and ramipril (Hope Study 2000), and statins (Haffner *et al.* 2000). Blood pressure should be measured at each visit. Hypertension often precedes microalbuminia in type 2 diabetes. Home and 24-hour blood pressure monitoring might provide useful information, exclude 'white coat' hypertension, and indicate loss of the normal nocturnal fall in blood pressure, which is an early sign of nephropathy (Jerums 2004).

Medication dose and/or dose interval adjustments and sometimes a change of medicines are required to renally excrete medicines when kidney function is compromised to avoid adverse events including hypoglycaemia because kidney disease affects the pharmacokinetic and pharmacodynamic processes. Inappropriate medicine regimens can lead to medicine-related adverse events and ineffective treatment (National Kidney Foundation Kidney Disease Outcomes Quality Initiative (K/DOQI) 2002). Older patients are at particular risk because of polypharmacy and age-related renal function decline. In addition, people should be asked about complementary and over-the-counter medicines as part of a regular systematic medicines review.

Relevant renally excreted medicines include digoxin, ACE, thiazide, loop and potassium-sparing diuretics, narcotics, antimicrobials, oral hypoglycaemic agents (OHAs), non-steroidal anti-inflammatory drugs (NSAIDs), statins and herbal medicines such as St. John's Wort and Gingko (Howes 2001; K/DOQI 2002). Long-acting sulphonylureas are usually contraindicated because of the risk of hypoglycaemia (K/DOQI 2002). The K/DOQI (2002) guidelines suggest metformin may not need to be completely avoided but recommend treatment should start with a low dose, slow titration and close monitoring for signs of lactic acidosis. Metformin should be discontinued temporarily during hypoxic conditions such as cardiac, liver and respiratory disease, other acute illnesses such as infection, and surgery and investigative procedures when the risk of lactic acidosis increases.

Retinopathy

Retinopathy consists of two broad categories: non-proliferative (NPDR) and proliferative retinopathy (PR). The most common abnormalities are microaneurysms, dot and blot haemorrhages and exudates on the retina. New capillaries grow on the retina and are fragile and prone to sudden bleeding. Macular oedema and vitreous haemorrhages occur gradually and are the main cause of visual loss. The risk of retinopathy increases with increasing duration of diabetes and the presence of renal disease. Retinopathy and renal disease often coexist, especially in type 1 diabetes. Prevention is important and includes controlling blood glucose and regular screening to detect and manage early changes. Laser therapy may be indicated to arrest the damage.

Neuropathy

Peripheral neuropathy

Peripheral neuropathy can have devastating consequences such as foot ulceration and amputation. Peripheral sensory neuropathy is the most common form of neuropathy, and is usually bilateral and symmetrical, and can be painful or painless with sensory loss. Reduced vision, dexterity and cognitive function often preclude older people from caring for their feet appropriately and need to be considered as risk factors for foot pathology and falls. These people need significant assistance with foot care. The discomfort caused by neuropathy is distressing, disturbs sleep and reduces quality of life.

Diabetes-related painful neuropathy is typically worse at night and the symptoms are similar in both feet. The condition may be acute or chronic and there is a wide range of symptoms including burning, deep aching, stabbing, electric or cramping type pain, or a feeling of extreme coldness in the feet. Allodynia, which is a painful response to a stimulus that is not usually painful such as wearing shoes or having the bedclothes on the feet at night, may also be present. If the pain starts during a period of poor glycaemic control or fluctuating blood glucose levels (such as when diabetes is first diagnosed or when changing treatments), it is likely to be related to diabetes and the symptoms usually resolve gradually as the glycaemic control stabilises.

If the pain has been present for more than 12 months it is less likely to resolve spontaneously and, if bothersome, can be treated. Some patients respond well to topical application of capsaicin-based creams such as Finalgon (nonivamide) applied for several weeks. Others may need systemic medicines to manage their pain. When medication is used, 'trial and error' is often necessary because no single treatment is effective or suitable for every patient. Often a combination of treatments works best and may be associated with fewer side effects than high doses of any one medicine. Medicines commonly used to treat neuropathic pain include tramadol, amitriptyline, venlafaxine XR, Neurontin (gabapentin), Lyrica (pregabalin) and oxycodone.

It is always important to assess nerve function in people with diabetes. Tests include ankle reflexes, ability to feel a 10-g monofilament, and vibratory perception to determine whether the person has intact sensation or is at increased risk of ulceration. If these tests are normal, the risk of ulceration is not increased because they are likely to feel pain if the foot is damaged and can be reassured. However, regular foot assessment every 6–12 months is still necessary because loss of sensation can occur in the future. If sensation is reduced, the patient requires advice on how to protect their feet and where to seek help if they develop a foot wound. Patients should always be made aware that maintaining good glycaemic control provides the best defence against loss of sensation.

Diabetic foot disease is a major reason for admission to hospital. Approximately 15% of people with diabetes develop a foot ulcer and foot ulcers are the most common cause of ulceration (Edmonds *et al.* 2004). Amputation rates vary among communities and countries and depend on available resources to detect and manage underlying causes. Management strategies include:

- regular foot examination (podiatrist, diabetes educator, endocrinologist, general practitioner);
- patient and health professional education about preventing, identifying and managing diabetic foot disease;
- self-care to reduce risks including foot self-care, maintaining a healthy lifestyle and controlling metabolic parameters; and
- coordinated multidisciplinary foot services to detect and manage the multifactorial components of diabetic foot pathology.

Autonomic neuropathy

Autonomic neuropathy is an important and under-recognised long-term complication of diabetes. It occurs in the majority of people with type 1 diabetes and many with type 2. Autonomic neuropathy refers to damage to the autonomic nerves, affects approximately 30% of people with diabetes, and the symptoms develop slowly (Aly and Weston 2002). Other conditions, such as Parkinson's disease, can also cause autonomic neuropathy.

Effects on the gastrointestinal tract (GIT) include slow peristalsis, reduced gastric motility and emptying, and reduced oesophagus and gall bladder motility (Aly and Weston 2002). Delayed gastric emptying can lead to oesophageal reflux and dysphagia. Gastroparesis occurs when the vagus nerve is affected and results in bloating, diarrhoea (often at night), and vomiting after food. GIT infections may occur as the undigested food ferments. In addition, blood glucose levels are affected, malnutrition may be present, and absorption of some oral medications may be changed.

If the cardiovascular nerves are affected, sympathetic arteriole tone is lost and postural hypotension occurs. Postural hypotension is more common in older people and is further aggravated by autonomic neuropathy. Effects on the bladder may lead to incomplete bladder emptying and significant volumes of residual urine, which predisposes the individual to urinary tract infections and incontinence, which can lead to acute metabolic disturbances such as diabetic ketoacidosis (DKA) and hyperosmolar non-ketonic coma (HONK). Prophylactic cranberry juice prevents bacteria sticking to the bladder wall and may reduce the incidence of urinary tract infections (Braun 2007).

Erectile dysfunction (ED) is common in men with diabetes (> 30%) and is often undiagnosed. Vascular disease as well as neuropathy contributes to ED. It can cause a significant psychological burden and depression, which further exacerbates the problem. Other causes of erectile dysfunction include: smoking, alcohol consumption, some medicines such as antihypertensive agents, increasing age, genital surgery, genital abnormalities, endocrine disorders and trauma. Management consists of taking a careful history including a sexual history, adopting a healthy lifestyle, medicine review, and managing blood glucose. Medicines such as the phosphodiesterase 5 (PDE 5) inhibitors, for example sildenafil, might be indicated for some men but are contraindicated if significant heart disease is present or the man is using nitrate medicines. Injections such as alprostadil and vacuum and implant devices are also available.

The effect on female sexuality is more difficult to define, and there may be differences between type 1 and type 2. Women with type 2 diabetes report more effects on their relationships, lower desire, arousal, and libido, and vaginal dryness. A careful sexual history and general assessment is important when deciding on a management strategy. Referral to a sexual counsellor might be beneficial in some cases.

Dental infection

Dental infection and caries are perhaps the 'forgotten' complication of diabetes, yet they are the most common infection in humans (Zoellner 2006). Dental infections such as abscesses and periodontitis are generally more severe in people with diabetes and contribute to poor control and inadequate dietary intake. Pain affects eating, and halitosis and dental caries can affect body image, self-esteem, and quality of life, and consequently glycaemic control.

If untreated, dental disease can lead to generalised sepsis and contribute to respiratory and cardiovascular problems (Taylor *et al.* 2000). Regular dental assessments should be part of the routine diabetes assessment and dental disease treated early.

Musculoskeletal effects

Hyperglycaemia is associated with a range of musculoskeletal problems that are not life-threatening but cause significant discomfort/pain and can affect quality of life, ability to exercise, and self-care. These include stiffened joints, cheiroarthropathy (prayer sign), Dupuytren's contracture, trigger finger, frozen shoulder, and carpel tunnel syndrome.

CASE DISCUSSION

> **Mr ZM**
>
> ***Mr ZM was referred to an endocrinologist by his GP at the request of the nursing home staff***
> Mr ZM is a 70-year-old man with dementia living in our nursing home. He has chronic poor control, and HbA_{1c} last time was 8%. He is on bronchodilators and steroids for chronic respiratory disease due to a history of heavy smoking.
> He has Mixtard 30/70, 26 units mane and 18 units with tea. He is relatively inactive but wanders a lot and lately has been having hypos because he does not eat much. Sometimes it is very difficult to test his blood glucose.
> Can you please advise about a care plan for him?

Diabetes educator

Older people with diabetes have twice the risk of developing dementia. Dementia and Alzheimer's disease are associated with under-nutrition and weight loss.

Mixtard insulin, regardless of the proportion (20/80, 30/70 or 50/50), is challenging for older people, especially those with dementia and unpredictable dietary intake. The Actrapid component of Mixtard 30/70 (the 30% part of the entire pre-mixed insulin) starts to work 30 minutes after administration, can peak in around 4 hours and lasts up to 8 hours. This means that if Mr ZM is given his morning insulin at 7.30 a.m., and eats breakfast at 8.00 a.m., the peak action of his insulin is just before lunch. If Mr ZM refuses to eat lunch, he is then at a very real risk of hypoglycaemia.

Often the symptoms of hypoglycaemia in people with dementia are quite different from other symptoms experienced by other people with diabetes. Behaviour can deteriorate with the person becoming uncooperative or aggressive. Refusal to allow staff to perform capillary blood glucose testing may occur while the blood glucose levels are falling. This same scenario could be repeated at bedtime when the evening meal Mixtard is peaking 4 hours after it is administered.

The peak action of the 70% intermediate-acting component of Mixtard occurs mid- to late afternoon following the breakfast dose and early morning from 2 a.m. onwards when it is administered with the evening meal. Reversal of hypoglycaemia resulting from intermediate-acting insulin can be more difficult compared to rapid or fast-acting insulin and could result in more severe symptoms and therefore more difficult to manage behavioural changes.

Mr ZM's HbA$_{1c}$ is 8%, and given his overall health, obtaining an improved HbA$_{1c}$ is not an objective; reducing hypoglycaemia and thereby maximising his safety and quality of life are the priorities. Two main issues need to be addressed: a review of his insulin regimen and developing strategies to increase carbohydrate intake when he refuses to eat.

Insulin

- Mr ZM could be changed to a twice-a-day bolus analog premix insulin such as Novomix30 or HumalogMix25. The rapid-acting components of these two insulins, unlike Mixtard 30/70, peak approximately 90 minutes after administration and last for 3–4 hours. Both insulins can be administered directly after food, which may be useful if Mr ZM refuses breakfast or dinner.
- Mixtard 30/70 could be ceased and a daily basal analog insulin such as Lantus prescribed. Lantus is a peakless insulin without the associated rises and falls in actions and could stabilise blood glucose levels more effectively, markedly reduce the incidence of hypoglycaemia, and have a positive effect on behaviour.

Diet strategies

- There are a variety of ways Mr ZM's carbohydrate intake could be increased throughout the day. If Mr ZM refuses a meal, offer a carbohydrate-containing drink such as milk, Sustagen or juice, or provide carbohydrate food that appeals to Mr ZM such as custard and fruit or ice cream and fruit.
- Encourage Mr ZM to eat carbohydrate foods with a lower glycaemic index (GI) as this can help to reduce the risk of low glucose excursions (see Chapter 4).
- Identify the foods Mr ZM usually eats. For example, does he always eat his breakfast? If so, another breakfast could be offered in place of the refused meals.
- Ask his family what foods he enjoys and encourage them to bring them in. Set up a specific box of food that the staff can offer Mr ZM when he refuses a meal. For example, small tins of baked beans and small packets of fruitcake.
- Provide food on a plate or bowl from home – this might help reduce Mr ZM's anxiety.
- Have food available in Mr ZM's room or the residents' lounge. For example, a plate of fruit pieces may allow Mr ZM to graze.

- Offer smaller and more frequent meals to maintain the blood glucose level more effectively.

Part of Mr ZM's management plan should include strategies to assist staff, including casual staff, to recognise the behavioural symptoms of hypoglycaemia, the strategies used to reduce its occurrence, and the treatment most likely to work for Mr ZM. Staff working as a team should try a variety of strategies and objectively document the degree of success.

Dietitian

I would ask the GP and the nursing home staff the following questions:

- How long has Mr ZM had diabetes?
- Does he have type 1 or type 2 diabetes?
- What is his understanding of diabetes and has there been a time when he self-managed the condition?
- Is he still smoking? If so, has he been offered smoking cessation advice?
- Are the staff in the nursing home adequately trained in evidence-based diabetes care and treatments?
- How severe is his dementia? Is he able to cope with diabetes self-management or should his diabetes be managed by the nursing home staff?
- Does he inject his own insulin? If not, who does it for him? Have the insulin technique and insulin sites been checked?
- It has been stated: 'he does not eat much.' Is that due to poor appetite or does his dementia prevent him from sitting at a table and concentrating on the task?
- Is his weight stable or is he losing weight? What is his BMI? Is he a healthy weight for his height?
- His diabetes control is poor. Is he symptomatic? For example, does he experience excessive thirst, frequent urination, infections, tiredness and fatigue?

I would also ask Mr ZM some questions depending on the severity of his dementia:

- Do you understand you have diabetes?
- Do you know what diabetes is?

- How much diabetes self-management are you willing to take on and how much are you willing to delegate?

I would provide self-management education if appropriate or refer Mr ZM to a diabetes educator. I would provide or ask the diabetes educator to provide education for the nursing home staff and advise them to:

- try changing his insulin from Mixtard 30 twice a day to a peakless long-acting insulin such as Lantus or Levemir;
- improve his glycaemic control if he is experiencing symptoms that affect his quality of life;
- monitor his blood glucose if Mr ZM is happy for them to do so;
- prepare finger foods and nutritional drinks to improve his nutritional intake.

Diabetes educator 2

Managing older people with diabetes, especially with dementia and in nursing homes, is very difficult. Changing to Lantus is likely to reduce his hypoglycaemia and may improve his glycaemic control (Janka *et al.* 2005). It may also reduce the care burden on the nursing staff. Improving his glycaemic control would be a first priority because it is very difficult to determine his mental status, degree of dementia, and cognitive and physical functioning when the blood glucose is erratic. If the hypoglycaemia is not addressed it can become chronic, more difficult to control and likely to result in falls and possibly trauma.

His life expectancy is another consideration and may depend on the type of dementia Mr ZM has. Discussing these issues with the family and explaining the factors affecting Mr ZM's erratic behaviour are both important. Achieving a lower HbA_{1c} might be less important then preventing hypoglycaemia and managing any diabetes complications and other comorbidities present. His wandering, hypoglycaemia, and agitation put him at significant risk of falling.

The wandering could be a consequence of his dementia, hypoglycaemia, pain, or stress. These factors need to be excluded or managed. The wandering constitutes activity and may need to be considered when deciding on his insulin doses. Oral pain could be contributing to his food refusal. A dental check is indicated to determine whether he has any oral problems affecting his ability to eat.

CASE DISCUSSION

> **Mrs MS**
>
> ***Mrs MS was referred by a diabetes educator in a rural area to a metropolitan diabetes educator***
>
> *History*
> Mrs MS is 45 and recently moved to Melbourne from NSW.
> She has not had any medical assessment for 18 months.
> She is married with two children aged 19 and 18 who live at home.
> She works as a mortgage manager in a local bank.
> Her periods have become irregular over the past year.
> She has no idea what her cholesterol level is.
> She smokes 'occasionally just socially'.
> Her father aged 79 has type 2 diabetes and hypertension.
> Her mother aged 75 has hypertension and dyslipidaemia.
> She has one brother who is overweight and is often tired.
>
> *Assessment*
> Overweight BMI 28 (normal < 25 kg/m² where practical)
> Waist circumference 32
> BP 146/84
> Urinalysis normal
> Laboratory blood glucose 8 mmol/L random
> Mixed lipidaemia-cholesterol 5.2 mmol/L
> Trigs 3.0 mmol/L
> HDL 0.8 mmol/L
> LDL 3.2 mmol/L
>
> *Twelve months later*
> Mrs MS presented again having not attended for any follow-up in the meantime.
> Her mother had an MI 6 months previously.
> She reports:
> Increasing fatigue
> Breathless at times
> Hot flushes
> Irritability
> Mostly high blood glucose levels
> Her HbA$_{1c}$ was 10.7% 6 months ago when she was seen by a locum doctor for the above symptoms.
> The locum told her to lose weight and get some exercise.

Diabetes educator

I would discuss her psychological status and determine whether she is under stress. I would check her insulin technique and take a history of episodes of DKA or hypoglycaemia and her home situation. I would review her insulin regimes and diet and make sure she is not having hypos and eating to compensate.

Diabetes educator 2

This woman is at significant and immediate risk of a cardiovascular event. She has elevated lipids especially her LDL, a family history of heart disease and dyslipidaemia, and her HbA_{1c} is very high, she is overweight, hypertensive, and she smokes. Her increasing fatigue and breathlessness could be due to her hyperglycaemia and weight, but an MI needs to be excluded. I would refer her for an ECG, troponins and cardiac enzymes and possibly a cardiac stress test.

She may be menopausal considering her hot flushes, irritability, and irregular periods. Hot flushes are the most commonly reported menopausal symptom and can affect sleep. The frequency and intensity vary greatly and continue for around 5 years but can persist for years, even the rest of the woman's life. Oestrogen and progesterone levels would be useful and could form the basis of a more detailed sexual history and management strategies. Other causes of fatigue and flushing need to be ruled out such as thyroid disease. Depression also needs to be considered and may be a result of and/or contribute to her inadequate self-care.

If her oestrogen and progesterone levels are low, a careful discussion about her treatment options are needed. Given her cardiac risk status, hormone replacement therapy (HRT) is probably contraindicated. Some of the newer antidepressants – selective serotonin reuptake inhibitors (SSRIs) and serotonin-norepinephrine reuptake inhibitors (SNRIs) reduce hot flushes in 60–70% of women (Eden 2006). Oral HRT may reduce total cholesterol (but not triglycerides) and may improve glycaemic control, but the long-term cardiovascular benefits are unknown and I would not recommend HRT for Mrs MS except in the very short term.

Women are also reluctant to use HRT since the publication of the Women's Health Initiative (WHI) study (2002) and many use complementary therapies including phytoestrogens such as soya, and herbal medicines such as Dong Quai (*Cimicifuga racemosa* or black cohosh), which, while there is some good evidence for its efficacy, can cause liver toxicity. Given Mrs MS's lipid levels she may have fatty liver, which might exclude its use. Although there is no evidence to support this statement I would not recommend she use it. I would refer her to an endocrinologist or gynaecologist for specific advice about her HRT options. She may also require a breast check and pap smear given her history of not attending regular follow-up care.

Smoking is known to exacerbate hot flushes and stopping smoking is a key strategy to alleviate the flushes and reduce her cardiovascular risks. She may benefit from a quit programme.

Mrs MS is also at risk of osteoporosis and a comprehensive nutritional review is needed. Exercise within her tolerance limits may help with her weight once her cardiovascular status is assessed and her bone strength is clarified. Exercises such as yoga and Tai Chi can improve muscle strength and flexibility. Avoiding hot, spicy foods and drinks and alcohol often helps reduce hot flushes. I would direct her to the Australian Menopause Society (or other relevant) website (*www.menopause.org.au*).

Endocrinologist

This woman has metabolic syndrome and needs a fasting glucose to clarify the elevated random glucose. Random glucose under 5.5 mmol/L does not reliably exclude diabetes but above these levels a fasting glucose is required. If the fasting glucose is at or above 5.5 mmol/L, a glucose tolerance test is required if significant risk factors for diabetes are present, which is the case with Mrs MS in view of her family history. However, other causes of this syndrome should be considered and tested for, if clinically indicated, such as Cushing's syndrome and, rarely, acromegaly. A thyroid function test would also be indicated with the weight gain. If no cause is found, a lifestyle modification programme similar to the Diabetes Prevention Programme has been shown to reduce the risk of progression to diabetes. At present the evidence is not sufficient to recommend preventive medication.

CASE DISCUSSION

Mr LOQ

Mr LOQ self-referred to a diabetes centre
I have a horrible burning feeling in my feet especially at night. I have had diabetes for a while and find it hard to stick to my diet and exercise because of this feeling.
     What can I do?
     Do you think vitamin B supplements will help?

Podiatrist

The burning feeling might be due to a condition called peripheral neuropathy. Peripheral neuropathy is one of the complications of diabetes that affects the nerves, especially to the feet. It is a very distressing condition and can be difficult to treat. Often the symptoms diminish over 12–18 months.

Different people respond to different treatments. Some treatments include medicines such as tricyclic antidepressants and quinidine. Other treatments include foot massage, applying a special film called Op-Site or food wrap over the painful areas, electrotherapy and acupuncture. Cold compresses made by soaking a washcloth in cold water, wringing out the excess water and applying the cloths over the area may help. The compresses can be repeated and used with other treatments.

Vitamin B is essential to healthy nerve function and some enzymes that enable carbohydrate to be used for energy. Supplements might help, especially if the diet is low in vitamin B and cannot be changed. It is found in cereals, bran, corn, wholemeal bread, soya products, nuts, seeds and vegemite. It is destroyed by cooking, so fresh foods are the best source.

Controlling your blood glucose, limiting alcohol intake and not smoking are also important. You should check your feet carefully because you most probably have some reduced sensation in your feet and are at risk of not recognising foot trauma. Footwear needs to be checked and advice about appropriate footwear and exercise is important.

Diabetes educator

Peripheral neuropathy is the most likely cause and the podiatrist has addressed the most important issues. However, there are other causes of the burning sensation Mr LOQ describes and these include hypothyroidism, spinal nerve compression, and musculoskeletal problems. These causes need to be excluded. His circulation needs to be checked. Often neuropathic pain is unrelenting and affects quality of life and causes depression, which need to be assessed and treated if necessary.

Complementary therapist

Although there is no scientific evidence to support the recommendation, I have found some people respond to high dose of vitamin B5 supplements at night before bed. It appears to take 1–2 weeks before symptom relief is noticed. I would not recommend people take vitamin B complex supplements at night because it can cause sleep disturbance in some people.

References

Aly N, Weston P (2002) Autonomic neuropathy in older people with diabetes mellitus. *Journal of Diabetic Nursing* 6(1): 10–15.

Australian and New Zealand Dialysis and Transplant Registry (ANZDATA) (2000) *ANZDATA Registry.* ANZDATA, Adelaide.

Australian Institute of Health and Welfare (AIHW) (2007) *Medicines for Cardiovascular Health.* Australian Government Report, May.

Bate KL, Jerums G (2003) Preventing complications of diabetes. *Medical Journal of Australia* 179: 498–503.

Bethel MA, Sloan FA, Belsky D *et al.* (2007) Longitudinal incidence and prevalence of adverse outcomes of diabetes mellitus in elderly patients. *Archives of Internal Medicine* 167(9): 921–927.

Braun L (2007) Cranberry Vaccinium macrocarpon. Journal of Complementary Medicine 6(3): 553–555.

Department of Health (2001) *Diabetes National Service Framework: Standards for Diabetes Services.* Department of Health, London.

de Zeeuw D, Remuzzi G, Parving H (2004) Albuminuria, a therapeutic target for cardiovascular protection in type 2 diabetic patients with nephropathy. *Circulation* 110(8): 921–927.

Diabetes Control and Complications Trial Research Group (DCCT) (1993) Effects of intensive insulin therapy on the development and progression of long-term complications of IDDM. *New England Journal of Medicine* 329: 977–986.

Dunning P, Martin M (1998) Seeking help for chest pain: NIDDM and non-diabetic responses to hypothetical scenarios. *Australian Journal of Advanced Nursing* 16 (1): 34–41.

Eden J (2006) Hormonal therapy and oral contraception in patients with diabetes. *Diabetes Management Journal* 14: 26.

Edmonds ME, Foster AVM, Sanders LJ (2004) *A Practical Manual of Diabetic Foot Care.* Blackwell Publishing, Massachusetts, pp 44–45, 48–50.

Goldberg R, Mellies M, Sacks F for the CARE investigators (1998) Cardiovascular events and their reduction with pravastatin in diabetes glucose-intolerant myocardial infarction survivors with average cholesterol levels. Subgroup analysis in the cholesterol and recurrent events (CARE) trial. *Circulation* 98: 1349–1357.

Haffner SM, Lehto S, Ronnemaa T *et al.* (2000) Mortality from coronary heart disease in subjects with type 2 diabetes and nondiabetic subjects with and without prior myocardial infarction. *New England Journal of Medicine* 339: 229–234.

Heart Outcomes Prevention Evaluation (HOPE) Study Investigators (2000) Effects of Ramipril on cardiovascular and microvascular outcomes in people with diabetes mellitus. *Lancet* 355: 253–259.

Hoogwerf B, Waness A, Cressman M *et al.* (1998) Effects of aggressive cholesterol-lowering and low-dose anticoagulation on clinical and angiographic outcomes in patients with diabetes. Post coronary artery bypass graft surgery. *Diabetes* 48: 1289–1294.

Hovind P (2005) Initiation, progression and remission of diabetic nephropathy. *Danish Medical Bulletin* 52(4): 119–142.

Howes L (2001) Dosage alterations in the elderly: importance of mild renal impairment. *Current Therapeutics* 42(7): 33–35.

Janka H, Plewe G, Busch K (2005) Combination of oral antidiabetic agents with basal insulin verses premixed insulin alone in elderly patients with type 2 diabetes. *Journal of the American Geriatrics Society* 55(2): 182–188.

Jerums G (2004) How should patients with microalbuminia and type 2 diabetes be treated? *Diabetes Management Journal* 8: 10–11.

Long-term Intervention with Pravastatin in Ischaemic Heart Disease (LIPID) Study Group (1998) Prevention of cardiovascular events and death with pravastatin in patients with coronary heart disease and a broad range of cholesterol levels. *New England Journal of Medicine* 339: 1349–1357.

Malmberg K, Norhammer A, Wedel H *et al.* (1999) Glycometabolic state at admission: important risk marker of mortality in conventionally treated patients with diabetes mellitus and acute myocardial infarction: long-term results from the diabetes and insulin-glucose infusion in acute myocardial infarction (DIGAMI) study. *Circulation* 99: 2626–2632.

Microalbuminuria Collaborative Study Group (1999) Predictors of the development of microalbuminuria in patients with type 1 diabetes mellitus: a seven year prospective study. *Diabetic Medicine* 16: 918–925.

Mosca L, Banka CL, Benjamin EJ *et al.* (2007) Evidence-based guidelines for cardiovascular disease prevention in women: 2007 update. *Circulation* 115(11): 1481–1501.

National Kidney Foundation (2002) Kidney disease outcomes quality initiative (K/DOQI). *American Journal of Kidney Diseases* 35(96): Suppl 2.

Parving HH, Lehnert H, Brochner-Mortensen J *et al.* (2001) The effect of irbesartan on the development of diabetic nephropathy in patients with type 2 diabetes. *New England Journal of Medicine* 345: 870–878.

Raskin P, Rosenstock J (1992) The genetics of diabetes complications. Blood glucose and genetic susceptibility. Chapter 53 in Albert K, DeFronzo R, Keen H *et al.* (eds) *International Textbook of Diabetes Mellitus.* John Wiley and Sons, Chichester.

Stuckey TD, Stone GW, Cox DA *et al.* (CADILLAC Team) (2005) Impact of stenting and abciximab in patients with diabetes mellitus undergoing primary angioplasty in acute myocardial infarction. *American Journal of Cardiology* 95: 1–7.

Taylor G, Loesche W, Terpenning M (2000) Impact of oral diseases on systemic health in the elderly: diabetes mellitus and aspiration pneumonia. *Journal of Public Health Dentistry* 60: 313–320.

UKPDS Group (1998) Intensive blood glucose control with sulphonylureas or insulin compared with conventional treatment and risk of complications in patients with type 2 diabetes (UKPDS 33). *Lancet* 352: 837–853.

Van de Veire N, de Winter O, Gir M *et al.* (2006) Fasting blood glucose levels are related to exercise capacity in patients with coronary artery disease. *American Heart Journal* 152(3): 486–492.

Zoellner H (2006) Oral problems in patients with diabetes. *Diabetes Management Journal* 14: 18–19.

Recommended reading

Apelqvist J, Bakker K, Van Houtum W *et al.* (2000) The international consensus and practical guidelines on the management and prevention of diabetic foot disease. *Diabetes/Metabolism Research and Review* 16(1): s84–s92.

International Diabetes Federation Consultative Section on Diabetes (2000) *Position Statement on Diabetes Education for People Who Are Blind or Visually Impaired.* International Diabetes Federation, Brussels, pp 62–72.

International Working Group on the Diabetic Foot (1999) *International Consensus on the Diabetic Foot.* International Working Group on the Diabetic Foot, The Netherlands.

National Kidney Foundation (2002) Clinical practice guidelines for nutrition in chronic renal failure. Kidney Outcome Quality Initiative (N/DOQI). *American Journal of Kidney Disease* 35 (96): Suppl 2.

Sorensen L, Molyneaux L, Yue D (2006) The relationship between pain, sensory loss and small nerve fibres in diabetes. *Diabetes Care* 29: 883–887.

UKPDS Group (1998) Intensive blood glucose control with sulphony-lureas or insulin compared with conventional treatment and risk of complications in patients with type 2 diabetes (UKPDS 33). *Lancet* 352: 837–853.

Chapter 8

Psychological issues and quality of life

> **Key points**
>
> - It is imperative that psychological, spiritual, and social aspects of an individual's life are considered when developing management plans.
> - These factors affect whether or not 'good' metabolic control is achieved.
> - Listening is a key health professional skill.
> - Health professionals need to understand themselves and their beliefs and attitudes.
> - Depression is common in people with diabetes and is often undiagnosed. Mental health assessment should be part of annual complication screening programmes.

Introduction

People respond to the diagnosis of diabetes depending on their overall resilience, psychological and social adjustment, and the availability of family support (Johnson 1980). Fitting diabetes into family life can be difficult and changes over time with increasing duration of diabetes and the complexity of the treatment regimen (Gardiner 1997). It is difficult to predict how an individual will react to the diagnosis of diabetes or the development of complications, but a number of common reactions have been described. These include grief, anger, loss, fear, shock, disbelief, and uncertainty, and denial is common. Many people associate the diagnosis with loss: loss of spontaneity and loss of choice and the good things in life. Others describe relief that they do not have 'something worse such as cancer'. Most understand the need to achieve 'tight control' – it is just not that easy to achieve, and even harder to maintain.

Achieving a balanced lifestyle and good quality of life (QoL) relevant to the individual is essential to the physical, psychological, and spiritual well-being of people with diabetes. The DAWN study (Rutherford *et al.* 2002) demonstrated the effects of stress on mental health and metabolic outcomes. People were more optimistic when they felt in control, whereas anxiety, problems coping, and burnout reduced well-being. Diabetes-related anxiety included fear of gaining weight, worsening of the disease, hypoglycaemia, and financial concerns. Type 2 respondents worried about needing to start insulin and developing complications.

Depression

Major depression occurs in one in five Australians and is increasingly associated with many common illnesses, including diabetes. A peak time for first diagnosis of depression occurs between the ages of 25 and 55. However, self-reported depressive symptoms and depression using depression rating tools appear to be associated with increased risk of developing diabetes in older people (Cardiovascular Health Study 2007). Observational studies also suggest that depression is an independent risk factor for death and managing the depression significantly reduces the risk (Gallo 2007). There are various types of depression: melancholic, non-melancholic, and clinical. An accurate diagnosis is necessary to ensure management is appropriate. Medicines may be necessary during depressive episodes.

Depression affects people's self-care ability and long-term health outcomes. People who are depressed are more likely to have inadequate self-care, present to the emergency department, require specialist intervention, and exhibit feelings of lowered self-worth and physical functioning (Ciechanowski *et al.* 2000). In addition, depression is predictive of type 2 diabetes. Goldney *et al.* (2004) suggested that at least 24% of Australians with diabetes are depressed but the depression remains undiagnosed in many cases. These findings are similar in other countries. There is a correlation between depression and poor diabetes control. There are many causes of depression (see Table 8.1).

Signs and symptoms of depression

Depression can be difficult to identify and is often recurrent. An episode of depression is defined as the presence of:

Table 8.1 Common causes of depression. Depression is multifaceted and common and impacts on diabetes self-care behaviour. All of these factors can lead to inadequate self-care, but the degree varies depending on the individual's social circumstances, personality, resilience, and coping ability.

Causes	Effects on self-care behaviours
A triggering event, e.g. the death of a spouse, diagnosis of diabetes	Poor adherence to dietary guidelines
Loneliness or isolation	Reduced dietary intake, even anorexia
Recurrent or constant pain, such as painful diabetic peripheral neuropathy	Poor compliance with medication regimens
	Weight gain due to inability to exercise
Urinary and/or faecal incontinence	Reduction or cessation of home blood glucose monitoring
Inability to perform activities of daily living (ADLs) due to chronic illness: diabetes, stroke, Parkinson's disease, rheumatoid arthritis, dependence on oxygen therapy	Reduced compliance with health appointments and complication screening
Weight gain as a result of diabetes medicines, such as sulphonylureas, thiazolidinediones, and insulin	Depression increases the risk of adverse diabetes-related outcomes (Black *et al.* 2003)
Loss of independence, which may be due to diabetes control, and can result in cancellation of a driver's licence	
Financial difficulties	
Sense of loss of control and reduced resilience	
Impaired cognition, or conversely depression may present as impaired cognition	
Adverse reactions to medicines such as antihypertensives (commonly used in people with diabetes), corticosteroids, non-steroidal agents, anti-Parkinson's disease drugs and analgesics	
Alcohol	
Diabetes-related complications such as impaired vision, need for enteral feeds and renal failure requiring renal dialysis	
Long duration of diabetes	

Table 8.1 (*Continued*)

Causes	Effects on self-care behaviours
Older age where motivation to adhere to management plan is reduced and there may be a common pathogenesis involving autonomic and sympathetic nerves (Black *et al.* 2003)	
Chronic hyperglycaemia	Tiredness
	Lethargy
	Dry mouth
	Thirst
	Polyuria
	Nocturia
	Weight loss
	Malnutrition

- a depressed mood, which is not influenced by circumstances and which is present for the entire duration of most days for at least 2 weeks;
- loss of interest or pleasure in activities or interests normally enjoyed; and
- lethargy.

In addition, at least four of the following may be evident:

- loss of self-esteem and self-confidence;
- inappropriate or excessive guilt feelings and, sometimes, false beliefs or delusions;
- recurrent thoughts of worthlessness and despair, which may precipitate thoughts of death or suicide;
- poor concentration and indecisiveness;
- agitation or significant reduction in activity levels;
- sleep disturbances; and/or
- changes in weight due to altered dietary habits (Gray *et al.* 2002).

Tools used to measure depression

The following validated screening tools are used to detect depression and reduced well-being:

- Geriatric Depression Score in older people who have high levels of depression, especially in residential care facilities (Gray *et al.* 2002).
- Diabetes Quality of Life Measure (DQoL).
- DMI 10.
- Cornell Depression Rating Scale.
- Medical Outcome Study Health Survey 36-item Short Form (SF-36).
- Health-Related Quality of Life Survey (HRQoL).
- Elderly Diabetes Impact Scales (EDIS) – Japan.
- Brief Case Finding for Depression (BCD).
- Hospital Anxiety and Depression Scale (HADS).
- Audit of Diabetes Dependent Quality of Life (ADDQoL).
- Beck Depression Inventory (BECK).

Psychological adaptation and maintaining a good quality of life depend on the individual's resilience, which refers to the ability to overcome adversity and not only rise above it, but also to thrive. Managing a chronic illness means integrating two distinct management paradigms – biomedical and psychosocial/spiritual – which need to be balanced to achieve holistic care. Importantly, health professionals must listen to their patients, including being aware of what is *not* said. Woodcock and Kinmonth (2001) compared nurses and patients to determine their agreement about patients' three main concerns and found only 36% agreement overall.

Quality of life

Over half of the people with type 2 diabetes on insulin report reduced quality of life. Insulin has a negative impact on quality of life, which is greater in younger people with long duration of diabetes from non-English speaking backgrounds (Rubin 2000; Davis *et al.* 2001). Men with type 2 diabetes self-report depression, disempowerment and perceived loss of control (Tun *et al.* 1990). The association between depression and insulin may be part of the mythology that insulin indicates severe disease or 'the end of the line' (Dunning and Martin 1997). More support and early explanations of the likely progression to insulin because of progressive beta cell failure are required for people with type 2 diabetes (see Chapter 2).

Quality of life is a highly subjective and multidimensional concept concerned with cognitive status, satisfaction, and emotional happiness. Poor quality of life is associated with neglecting self-care including medicines, and may predict an individual's capacity for self-care (Cox and Gonder-Frederick 1992).

Factors that determine QoL fall into four main categories:

(1) *Medical* – diabetes type, treatment regimen, level of metabolic control, and the presence of complications. The severity of complications reduces the QoL. Yet, diabetes and complications can be positive triggers for change. However, level of glycaemic control does not necessarily relate to QoL (Testa *et al.* 1998), whereas symptoms and nutritional status in older people do (Van der Does *et al.* 1996; Maaravi *et al.* 2000).

(2) *Cognitive* – acute and chronic blood glucose control and neuropsychological changes can reduce the QoL for the person with diabetes and his or her family.

(3) *Beliefs and attitudes* – self-efficacy, mastery, resilience, locus of control, meaningfulness, and social support. People with good support have better QoL and less depression. Empowerment strategies and improving an individual's sense of being in control improves his or her QoL.

(4) *Demographic* – gender, education level, ethnicity, culture, age, and financial security.

It is important to use standardised, validated QoL tools when comparing different individuals, especially for research purposes. Determining the individual's QoL issues (patient-generated QoL) and measuring them periodically may be a more useful way to gauge an individual's well-being (Jenkinson and McGee 1998). Developing a therapeutic relationship with the individual, active listening, and recognising that diabetes may not always be the top priority in the person's life are all important. Strategies to help people cope with stress and education to help them develop problem-solving skills are important management strategies.

CASE DISCUSSION

Mrs MJ

Mrs MJ was referred to a diabetes centre by her GP
Mrs MJ, a 60-year-old woman with type 2 diabetes since 2000, presents with:
Random blood glucose 21.9 mmol/L
Fasting glucose 17.8 mmol/L
HbA$_{1c}$ 14.3%. Her HbA$_{1c}$ has steadily increased over the past 18 months
Total cholesterol 4.1
HDL 1.76
LDL 2.0

Trigs 0.8
BP 140/80.
I have been suggesting she start insulin for the past 12 months but Mrs MJ repeatedly refuses insulin.

Current medications

Diamicron (gliclazide)	2 mg	BD
Atenolol	2.5 mg	BD
Frusemide	40 mg	
Actos (pioglitazone)	45 mg	
Ramipril	5 mg	BD
Simvastatin	40 mg	BD
Aspirin	$1/_2$ tablet	daily

She was on Daonil in the past but said it caused headaches and chest pain and stopped taking it, at which point she was commenced on Diamicron.

She refuses to take metformin because it gives her diarrhoea.

Her diet is not ideal (she loves chocolate) and she does not exercise.

Weight 60.9 kg (steady).

She has known ischaemic heart disease, no other complications detected.

Left cataract surgery in 2000 and has had a retinal haemorrhage.

She varies her Diamicron dose or does not take it according to how she feels and her BGLs.

Mrs MJ has been commenced on many medicines for diabetes and other diseases but reports 'side effects' shortly after starting each one, e.g. Plaquenil (hydroxychloroquine) 'causes headaches'. This was prescribed for a long-standing history of polymorphous light eruption. She has regular dermatology appointments for this condition.

Psychologist

Mrs MJ is understandably, like many other individuals, reluctant to use insulin, an issue that is referred to by some authors as 'psychological insulin resistance'. It is important to note that this is not injection or needle phobia. The published literature indicates that needle phobia is rare, less than 1% of people with diabetes, and usually only found in individuals who have other concurrent phobias (Mollema *et al.* 2001). It is important to acknowledge that most people feel apprehensive about starting insulin and to identify the origins of such apprehension. Undoubtedly, it partly arises from fear about injections generally, because many people associate injections with needles into a muscle or blood vessel with pain and are worried that insulin injections will be painful.

However, the patient's anxiety about insulin is not solely related to fear of pain. Health care professionals frequently, although unintentionally, give the message that people should be afraid of insulin and that it should be avoided if possible. For example, at diagnosis a health professional may say: '*Don't worry, you do not have the type of diabetes that needs insulin,*' which subtly conveys the message that insulin is something to be worried about. Later in the life of the person with diabetes, it is relatively common to hear health professionals say: '*If we do not get your blood glucose levels down we are going to have to put you on to insulin.*' When insulin (or anything else) is used as a threat to motivate change the implication is the person should be scared (Hunt *et al.* 1997; Lauritzen and Scott 2001). Taking the time to enquire about Mrs MJ's concerns about insulin, taking care to elicit all her concerns, talking through each one with her are all vital. Supporting her to insert a needle into herself may help overcome her fear that the injection will be painful.

The information provided in the referral letter suggests a more general additional challenge, with her history of trialling different medications, reporting side effects to most of them, and her history of discontinuing treatment. It is also noteworthy that she only takes her Diamicron according to what she 'feels' her blood glucose levels are, which suggests she only takes her medication when she is symptomatic. Therefore, she may make inappropriate decisions because people do not accurately predict their blood glucose levels. However, these actions are not unusual behaviours by people with diabetes (Murphy and Kinmonth 1995) and people with hypertension (Baumann and Leventhal 1985), which suggests Mrs MJ may vary her antihypertensive medication doses as well.

There is a great deal of literature about people's medication and illnesses beliefs. A common feature in the literature is that people struggle to understand their health condition, and take it seriously, if they do not have some kind of concrete evidence of its existence such as a sign or symptom they can relate to. Therefore, when people take medication, they generally expect to experience an alleviation of some indicator of their condition, and frequently manage their illness accordingly. Unfortunately, many symptoms are incorrectly attributed and sometimes interpreted as a medicine-related side effect.

So how can we address these potential factors and incorporate Mrs MJ's obvious attention to her health and wellness into a management plan? The first step is to identify:

- her diabetes beliefs;
- what she considers to be the problem with her body;
- what she thinks caused the problem;
- her understanding of the different treatments she has tried or is using and their mode of action; and
- how she tells what her blood glucose levels are (high or low).

Once you understand her knowledge of and beliefs about her diabetes, you are in a better position to identify and address misconceptions. If you do identify a misconception it is important to enquire about the factors and/or experiences that led to her beliefs. Only when you understand her and her beliefs, will you be able to provide effective education and support. So take time to listen before taking time to explain.

Endocrinologist

This woman needs insulin therapy *and* intensive education about the fact that her feelings are not a good guide to her blood glucose levels, which is a common misconception or excuse. It would be useful to regularly download her meter information and confront her with this evidence. It has been found to be useful, with psychological insulin resistance, to emphasise:

- insulin is the most powerful drug we have for controlling glucose;
- insulin injections hurt less than fingerpricks;
- most people have more energy when commenced on insulin because of improvement in their glucose levels; and
- starting insulin does not lock her in to insulin therapy – if she stops it, she will be no worse off than before.

A useful strategy is to offer a trial of insulin for 1 month and if Mrs MJ does not feel much better, she can stop the therapy. Her beliefs and perceptions about insulin need to be explored, because false beliefs about it are sometimes a cause of insulin refusal.

Diabetes educator

I agree with the psychologist's insightful comments and these issues need to be addressed before the physical issues such as the high HbA_{1c} and lipids can be corrected. Polymorphous light eruption (PMLE) has a substantial psychological and social impact, especially in women (Richards *et al.* 2007), which could compound Mrs MJ's diabetes-related anxieties.

Mrs MJ clearly does need insulin. The slow progressive nature of type 2 diabetes may never have been explained to her and she may blame herself for 'failing' or feel guilty that she has not managed to control her diabetes despite 'listening' to her body. Given her PMLE insulin may represent another burden to bear. Explaining what is happening to her body may help her accept insulin as a necessary replacement rather than a punishment, especially if she can stop her oral medicines. It is important that she is well informed about the risks and benefits of not starting insulin and that health professionals listen to her reasons for not wanting insulin.

Health professionals commonly focus on the negative aspects of a situation, as the psychologist implied. Focusing on the positive aspects of insulin is important. Mrs MJ has probably been told repeatedly that she needs insulin to prevent complications (she already has several and a long-standing intercurrent illness). I would ask her to think about just one positive thing about insulin and to write it down so we could discuss it at her next appointment. Commencing insulin for people like Mrs MJ is a slow process and health professionals need to allow time, and respect her opinion. It is also worth considering that a patient 'not listening' could be a cue to the health professional to change their approach.

Medicine side effects are more common than health professionals realise and are a common reason for stopping medicines. Health professionals often refer to 'mild side effects' – they may be far from mild to the person experiencing them. Mrs MJ may have been commenced on a high dose of metformin initially and it may well have caused diarrhoea or other gastrointestinal symptoms. Combining metformin and insulin in people with type 2 diabetes is often effective and it would be worth explaining these issues to Mrs MJ in the hope she might agree to try metformin again at low doses and gradually increase to tolerance.

However, given her eye disease and macrovascular disease she probably also has renal damage and oral glucose-lowering agents may be contraindicated. Her renal status needs to be established as part of the decision-making process. She was prescribed Plaquenil for her PMLE. Retinopathy is an absolute contraindication to Plaquenil. Given the fact that she has had a retinal haemorrhage alternative treatments may be required. I would suggest the GP refers her to her dermatologist and advises him or her about the retinal haemorrhage.

If she does agree to take insulin, it would be very important not to cause hypoglycaemia, and to make the regimen as simple as possible. A long-acting analogue is the insulin of choice. Mrs MJ has known cardiovascular disease and the chest pain may have occurred coincidentally when she took Daonil, but she may have been experiencing hypoglycaemia, which could cause the headaches she described. It is not clear whether her chest pain was investigated to exclude angina or MI and this should be considered. She is also on a statin, which may cause muscle aches, which Mrs MJ could mistake for chest pain.

She is also on Actos, which could be causing oedema and discomfort and may be contraindicated depending on her degree of heart disease (see Chapter 5).

Her love of chocolate could be used positively. Small amounts of dark chocolate have a similar effect on platelets as aspirin (Faraday 2006) and could be included in her diet. A dietary review would be useful. Mrs MJ was probably told to wear protective clothing when she is outside and is most likely deficient in vitamin D, which increases her risk of osteoporosis.

Considering her age and blood glucose control and intercurrent illnesses, it is important to ensure she has influenza and pneumonia vaccinations each year and any grandchildren should also be vaccinated if they regularly come into contact with her.

I would enquire into her social situation, which may affect her decisions. She could be depressed and her mood and cognitive functioning need to be assessed. Given her random blood glucose level of 21.9 mmol/L it is likely that is also contributing to her lethargy and lowered mood and may affect her ability to make decisions. These factors, in addition to those raised by the psychologist, may affect her medicine-related decision-making.

Podiatrist

Mrs MJ's feet need to be assessed to determine whether she is at risk of foot ulcers given her history of suboptimal glucose control and the presence of micro- and macrovascular disease. Details about foot care and assessment can be found in Chapter 7.

CASE DISCUSSION

Mrs KB

Mrs KB was referred to an endocrinologist by her GP
Thank you for advising about this 59-year-old woman with type 2 diabetes. She has all the risk factors for cardiovascular disease, has early retinopathy and has been admitted several times to stabilise her diabetes.

   She is on very large doses of insulin; current dose 120 units/day overall.
   Her HbA$_{1c}$ at the moment is 16%.
   BMI 35 kg/m^2.
   She has seen both the dietitian and diabetes educator but does not listen to a thing they say.
   What to do?

Psychologist

This brief letter gives little to go on, but the last statement is a common complaint of many health care professionals and warrants consideration. The assertion is that Mrs KB 'does not listen to a thing they say'. The question I would ask is: How do the diabetes educator and dietitian know she does not listen? It is worth noting that both patient and professional recall of consultations is more inaccurate than accurate, with many professionals recalling making recommendations in consultations that were never actually made (Skinner *et al.* 2007). What these health professionals probably mean is that they do not see any evidence that Mrs KB changes her behaviour, because her HbA$_{1c}$ is still high and her BMI does not reduce. So health professionals feel they are not being listened to.

Assuming the diabetes educator gives very clear information and has checked that Mrs KB understands the information, the factors that prevent Mrs KB from following the advice given need to be identified. In reality, she probably has more reasons for not following the advice than reasons to follow it. One issue to consider is how the messages Mrs KB receives from a range of health professionals could differ and influence her self-management behaviours. It is common for health professionals to point out to people with type 2 diabetes how serious the complications of diabetes are, to reiterate that they will undoubtedly get complications if they do not control their diabetes, and encourage them to adopt a range of behaviour changes in order to control their diabetes. The health professionals' behaviours are largely based on the premise that the more serious and at-risk an individual perceives him- or herself to be, the more likely he/she is to take action, and that most people underestimate their risk.

Research suggests that people with type 2 diabetes tend to substantially overestimate their risk of heart disease and strokes in the next 10 years by about 20% (Frijling *et al.* 2004; Asimokopoulou *et al.* 2006). These findings differ from the widely held belief that people exhibit 'optimistic bias' and underestimate their risk. However, research, predominantly with student samples but also in the patient and genetic counselling literature, consistently shows that people overestimate risk (Butow *et al.* 2003). Such pessimistic bias would not necessarily be a problem if the individual were able to take the necessary actions to reduce the risk.

Unfortunately, in combination with low self-efficacy beliefs, high perceptions of risk are unlikely to motivate behaviour change. People with diabetes often learn through the media, multiple conversations with multiple health care professionals, and from family and friends, a long list of things they need to do to reduce their risk of getting complications. These messages include reduce the amount you eat, increase your fruit and vegetable consumption, reduce the amount of fat you eat, reduce the amount of saturated fat you eat, eat more fibre, reduce your salt intake, increase your levels of physical activity, stop smoking, reduce the amount of sugar in your diet, reduce the glycaemic index of the food you eat, eat more oily fish, take your medication, monitor your blood glucose levels. Long lists of 'do and do not' can be so overwhelming that people feel unable to do all of these things and rationalise 'if I can't do all of that, what's the point,' and do not do anything.

So how could we help Mrs KB? First, we need to help her understand her personal risks: that is personalise the risk information for her. There are plenty of risk engines available free to all health care professionals to facilitate this. These risk engines can also be used to help Mrs KB understand the impact of each different risk factor (BMI, HbA_{1c}, lipids, hypertension) on her overall risks. The information can be used to negotiate with Mrs KB to focus on one risk factor and help her identify the strategies she can use to reduce that risk factor.

Focusing on one thing at a time and having the patient select the risk factor they want to focus on and the ways to address it is more likely to be successful. She can be involved in developing an initial plan, focusing on one or two behaviours initially and have a clear strategy for deciding whether the changes she makes help her to reduce the risk factor. There is an old, very relevant Chinese proverb that suits Mrs KB's situation: 'a thousand mile journey begins with a single step.'

Diabetes educator

I agree with the strategy outlined by the psychologist. Mrs KB clearly has insulin resistance, which needs to be investigated. Insulin resistance is a feature of type 2 diabetes and is multifactorial in nature. Genetic makeup and lifestyle factors such as inappropriate diet and lack of exercise play a role.

However, it is important to determine whether Mrs KB's weight gain is due to lifestyle or whether she has an underlying endocrine disorder or is taking any medicines that compound the lifestyle risk factors. Her cardiovascular risk is a concern and needs to be investigated. Her lipid levels are not provided but they are probably high given her blood glucose level. Infection needs to be ruled out.

A list of medicines was not provided. It is important to review the medicines she is taking, some of which could be contributing to her weight. It would be worth checking her insulin administration technique to ensure she is actually taking the prescribed doses, and checking her injection sites.

A possible strategy is to admit Mrs KB and give her an insulin infusion to reduce the blood glucose and correct her lipids and then commence insulin again. If she is not on insulin analogues, they could be commenced. Bariatric surgery might be considered. I would refer her to an endocrinologist to ensure she does not have an underlying endocrine disorder.

Endocrinologist

As well as the considerations outlined by the psychologist, medical causes of Mrs KB's insulin resistance need to be excluded, which would include:

- microurine culture and chest X-ray to exclude occult sepsis;
- insulin-like growth factor 1 (IGF-1) to exclude acromegaly;
- 24-hour urinary free cortisol to exclude Cushing's syndrome; and
- thyroid function tests to exclude hyper- or hypothyroidism.

With more severe insulin resistance, insulin receptor antibodies could be measured.

Podiatrist

This woman's macro and microvascular risk profile and non-compliance put her at risk of foot ulcers. She needs a thorough foot assessment and most probably foot self-care education.

CASE DISCUSSION

Mrs AV

Mrs AV was referred to the endocrinologist for 'assessment and advice' by her GP

Mrs AV is a 68-year-old Greek-speaking woman with type 2 diabetes of 20 years' duration. She has a history of Bell's palsy, osteoarthritis, glaucoma, blindness in her right eye, 'progressive' anaemia of unknown origin, and *Helicobacter pylori.*

Her most recent fasting blood glucose was 16.8 mmol/L.

Weight 70.8 kg

Current medications

Amitriptyline	10 g	nocte
Diamicron (gliclazide)	80 mg	BD
Metformin	1 g	TDS
Tritace (ramipril)	dose and dose frequency not indicated in notes	
Zantac (ranitidine)	20 mg/day	
Ramipril	5 mg/day	

Biochemistry results

Random blood glucose	25 mmol/L
HbA$_{1c}$	7.5%
Haemoglobin	10.4 (normal 11.5–16.5)
Na	134 (normal 135–145)
K$^+$	5.7 (normal 3.5–5.0)
Urea	13.1 (normal 2.5–6.4)
Creatinine	160 (normal 50–100)

On physical examination

She was very symptomatic, including nocturia 4–5 times per night

Disturbed sleep

No oedema

BP 160/80

She appears to be depressed.

Psychologist

This woman is clearly having a tough time of things, with multiple comorbidities for which she is on multiple medications. It is no surprise that her sleep is disturbed and she appears depressed. These two issues are probably related (disturbed sleep being a symptom of depression) and could be having a substantial impact on her health. The evidence is now considered relatively unequivocal, in that:

- depression is about 1.8 times more common in people with type 2 diabetes than in the general population (Ali *et al.* 2006);
- depression is predictive of heart disease (Bunker *et al.* 2003); and
- depression is associated with elevated blood glucose and complications (de Groot *et al.* 2001).

The good news is that the research also indicates that treating depression improves people's mood and can help improve metabolic outcomes

(Lustman *et al.* 2000), and the extra cost of treating depression is off-set by the reduction in other health care costs (Katon *et al.* 2006).

Therefore, exploring Mrs AV's emotional well-being is a good place to start and could be undertaken using a validated question-naire. However, questionnaires do not replace attentive listening and asking Mrs AV how she feels emotionally because symptoms of depression can be similar to those of other medical conditions. As well as assessing for depressed mood, we need to find out why she lacks positive emotions and why she has lost interest in things she used to find interesting.

If the health professional and Mrs AV agree that she is depressed, there are a number of options available to help her. These include medication, which can be discussed, but should not be forced. The main reason to consider medication is that symptom relief is rapid, usually 2–3 weeks after starting treatment. Once her mood and inter-est in things improve, psychological therapies can be included and it will be easier for her to participate in such therapies, which increases their effectiveness.

It is worth noting that Mrs AV is already on amitriptyline 10 g nocte, but it is not clear from the referral whether it was prescribed for depression or to treat painful peripheral neuropathy. The prescribed dose is lower than would be usual for depression; therefore it may be worth considering increasing the dose to levels shown to be effective in depression, which would avoid adding another medicine to her regi-men. If she cannot tolerate the common side effects at higher doses, other antidepressant medications should be considered. It is also important to monitor the effect of the medication and encourage Mrs AV to keep taking it for at least 3 weeks before deciding whether it is helping. It is common for people to have to try a second or third antidepressant before they find the one that works for them.

If Mrs AV wishes to undertake a psychological therapy, cognitive behaviour therapy (CBT) has a good evidence base. A trained psychol-ogist or cognitive therapist should undertake CBT. However, finding a psychologist is often difficult and expensive and there may be a long waiting list. Another option to consider is bibliotherapy. There are a number of well-designed self-help books available. Bibliotherapy is usually based on CBT and shows promising results. The main prob-lems with bibliotherapy is that people who are depressed have low motivation levels, and will struggle to do the homework that is key to its effectiveness.

Regular appointments or telephone calls can be an effective way to support Mrs AV, to help maintain her motivation and monitor her progress.

Endocrinologist

The HbA_{1c} results may not be accurate in patients with anaemia, as evidenced here by the lack of concordance with the patient's glucose results. This is a critical point to address because increasingly patients themselves as well as doctors are too focused on HbA_{1c} to the exclusion of doing enough of their own glucose monitoring. A pitfall seen in Mediterranean-origin patients is thalassaemia minor, which can result in errors in the HbA_{1c} assay through either increased red blood cell turnover and false low results, or cross reactivity of hepatic blood flow (HBF) in the assay with high-pressure liquid chromatography (HPLC)-based methods. Fructosamine estimation is the preferred method in theses cases. For this woman I would recommend haemoglobin electrophoresis to investigate whether she has thalassaemia.

Diabetes educator

There is no indication whether Mrs AV speaks and understands English although we are told she is Greek-speaking. She may need an interpreter, particularly to discuss possible depression. It is not desirable to use family to interpret in such circumstances. If she has mild depression rather than severe depression, St John's Wort may be worth considering if there are no likely medicine interactions.

In addition to the obvious need to determine her mental status and ensure it is adequately treated and monitored, her physical condition needs to be considered. She appears to have elevated creatinine and urea, which could indicate renal disease, which is likely, given her long duration of diabetes. If so, her medications may need to be reviewed and insulin may be simpler for her to manage.

Her blood pressure is high and needs to be investigated and treated given her cardiovascular risks. Her haemoglobin is slightly below normal. Her HbA_{1c} is acceptable considering her comorbidities. However, it may be lower than actual because of her anaemia (see Chapter 2). Mrs AV is Greek and may have a haemoglobinopathy such as thalassaemia and it might be worth having a fructosamine level measured, given that she is 'very symptomatic.' Mrs AV illustrates some of the pitfalls of using HbA_{1c} as the only indicator of metabolic control (Tran *et al.* 2004).

Anaemia may also be contributing to her tiredness, and folate supplements may be indicated. If she does not have thalassaemia (not helped by iron) she might also require iron supplements. Bone densitometry is indicated.

Her symptoms may be due to hyperglycaemia but a urinary tract infection needs to be excluded, so a micro urine and culture is indicated. Nocturia is likely to be disturbing her sleep and could exacerbate her lowered mood.

References

Ali S, Stone M, Peters J *et al.* (2006) The prevalence of comorbid depression in adults with type 2 diabetes: a systematic review and meta-analysis. *Diabetic Medicine* 23: 1165–1173.

Asimokopoulou K, Fox C, Marsh S *et al.* (2007) Unrealistic pessimism about risk of coronary heart disease and stroke in patients with type 2 diabetes. *Diabetic Medicine* 24(1): 30–121.

Baumann LJ, Leventhal H (1985) 'I can tell when my blood pressure is up, can't I?' *Health Psychology* 4(3): 203–218.

Bunker SJ, Colquhoun DM, Esler MD *et al.* (2003) 'Stress' and coronary heart disease: psychosocial risk factors. *Medical Journal of Australia* 178(6): 272–276.

Butow PN, Lobb EA, Meiser B *et al.* (2003) Psychological outcomes and risk perception after genetic testing and counselling in breast cancer: a systematic review. *Medical Journal of Australia* 178(2): 77–81.

Cardiovascular Health Study (CGS) (2007) Depressive symptoms may be linked to risk for incident diabetes in older adults. *Archives of Internal Medicine* 167: 802–807.

Ciechanowski P, Katon W, Russo W (2000) Impact of depressive symptoms on adherence, function and costs. *Archives of Internal Medicine* 160: 3278–3285.

Cox D, Gonder-Frederick L (1992) Major developments in behavioural diabetes research. *Journal of Consulting Clinical Psychologists* 60: 628–638.

Davis T, Clifford R, Davis W (2001) Effect of insulin therapy on quality of life in type 2 diabetes mellitus: the Fremantle diabetes study. *Diabetes Research and Clinical Practice* 52: 63–67.

de Groot M, Anderson R, Freedland K *et al.* (2001) Association of depression and diabetes complications: a meta-analysis. *Psychosomatic Medicine* 263: 619–630.

Dunning P, Martin M (1997) Using a focus group to explore perceptions of diabetes severity. *Practical Diabetes International* 14(7): 185–188.

Faraday (2006) Chocolate has antithrombotic effects similar to aspirin. *American Heart Association Scientific Sessions*, Chicago, November 14, Abstract 4101.

Frijling B, Lobo C, Keus I *et al.* (2004) Perceptions of cardiovascular risk among patients with hypertension or diabetes. *Patient Education and Counselling* 52: 47–53.

Gallo J (2007) Depression care management may reduce mortality in older adults. *Archives of Internal Medicine* 146: 689–698.

Gardiner P (1997) Social and psychological implications of diabetes mellitus for a group of adolescents. *Practical Diabetes International* 14(2): 43–46.

Goldney R, Phillips P, Fisher L *et al.* (2004) Diabetes, depression and quality of life. *Diabetes Care* 27: 1066–1067.

Gray L, Woodward M, Scholes R *et al.* (2002) *Geriatric Medicine* (2nd edn). Ausmed Publications, Melbourne.

Hunt L, Valenzuela M, Pugh J (1997) NIDDM patients' fears and hopes about insulin therapy: the basis of patient reluctance. *Diabetes Care* 20: 292–298.

Jenkinson C, McGee H (1998) *Health Status Measurement: A Brief but Critical Introduction.* Radcliffe Medical Press, Oxford, pp 61–63.

Johnson S (1980) Psychosocial factors in juvenile diabetes. *Journal of Health Psychology* 9: 737–749.

Katon W, Unutzer J, Fan MY *et al.* (2006) Cost-effectiveness and net benefit of enhanced treatment of depression for older adults with diabetes and depression. *Diabetes Care* 29(2): 265–270.

Lauritzen T, Scott A (2001) Barriers to insulin therapy in type 2 diabetes: a qualitative focus group research among patients, GPs and diabetologists. *European Union of General Practitioners Clinical Journal* 1(1): 36–44.

Lustman P, Freedland K, Griffith L *et al.* (2000) Fluoxetine for depression in diabetes. A randomized double-blind placebo-controlled trial. *Diabetes Care* 23: 618–623.

Maaravi Y, Berry E, Ginsberg G *et al.* (2000) Nutrition and quality of life in the aged: Jerusalem 70-year-olds, longitudinal study. *Aging Clinical Experience* 12(3): 173–179.

Mollema ED, Snoek FJ, Heine RJ *et al.* (2001) Phobia of self-injecting and self-testing in insulin-treated diabetes patients: opportunities for screening. *Diabetic Medicine* 18(8): 671–674.

Murphy E, Kinmonth A (1995) No symptoms, no problem? Patients' understandings of non-insulin dependent diabetes. *Family Practice* 12: 184–192.

Richards H, Ling T, Evangelou G *et al.* (2007) Psychological polymorphous light eruption and its relationship to patients' beliefs about their condition. *Dermatology* 56(3): 426–431.

Rubin R (2000) Diabetes and quality of life. From research to practice. *Diabetes Spectrum* 13: 21.

Rutherford A, Wright E, Hussain Z *et al.* (Australasian DAWN Committee) (2004) *DAWN (Diabetes Attitudes, Wishes and Needs): The Australasian Experience*. Novo Nordisk Australasia, Sydney.

Sinclair J, Finucane P (2001) *Diabetes in Old Age*. John Wiley and Sons, Chichester.

Skinner TC, Barnard K, Cradock S *et al.* (2007) Patient and professional accuracy of recalled treatment decisions in outpatient consultations. *Diabetic Medicine* 24(5): 557–560.

Testa MA, Simonson DC, Turner RR (1998) Valuing quality of life and improvements in glycaemic control in people with type 2 diabetes. *Diabetes Care* 21(3): c44–c52.

Tran H, Silva D, Petrovsky N (2004) Case study: potential pitfalls of using hemoglobin A_{1c} as the sole measure of glycaemic control. *Clinical Diabetes* 22: 141–143.

Tun P, Nathan D, Perlminter L (1990) Cognitive and affective disorders in elderly diabetics. *Clinical Geriatric Medicine* 6: 731–746.

Woodcock A, Kinmonth AL (2001) Patient concerns in their first year with type 2 diabetes: patient and practice nurse views. *Patient Education and Counselling* 242(3): 257–270.

Recommended reading

Diabetes Australia and the Royal Australian College of General Practitioners (RACGP) (2006) *Diabetes Management in General Practice 2005–2006*. RACGP, South Melbourne.

Diabetes Control and Complications Trial (DCCT) Research Group (1993) Influence of intensive diabetes treatment on quality of life outcomes in the DCCT. *Diabetes Care* 19: 195–203.

Centre for Mental Health Research, Australian National University. MoodGYM program (www.blackdoginstitute.org.au/index.cfm).

Padesky C, Greenberger D (1995) *Mind Over Mood: Change How You Feel by Changing the Way You Think*. Guilford, New York.

Snoek F, Skinner C (2000) *Psychology in Diabetes Care*. John Wiley and Sons, Chichester.

Snoek F, Pouwer F, Welch GW (2000) Diabetes-related emotional distress in Dutch and US diabetic patients: cross-cultural validity of the problem areas in diabetes scale. *Diabetes Care* 23: 1305–1309.

Tanner S, Ball J (1989) *Beating the Blues: A Self-Help Approach to Overcoming Depression*. Doubleday, New York.

Chapter 9

Diabetes education

Key points

- Diabetes education is a lifelong process and is essential to best practice diabetes management.
- Understanding the individual's learning style and health goals is essential to providing effective diabetes education.
- Education needs change over time, as the disease progresses, management changes, and complications develop.
- Counselling is an essential aspect of diabetes education.

Introduction

Despite sophisticated modern diabetes management methods, medications and technological advances many people with diabetes do not reach optimal metabolic targets, complication rates are still high, and many people have knowledge deficits (Tibbetts 2006). Most evidence-based guidelines document the central role of diabetes education, but provide limited guidance about the frequency, quality and standards required of diabetes education apart from the International Diabetes Federation (IDF) Consultative Section on Diabetes Education (DECS) guidelines. There is also little information about which aspects of education programmes produce the best outcomes. These issues are complex and multifactorial. Educators' skills and attitudes – as well as their knowledge and ability to adapt their teaching style to the individual's leaning style – all play a part.

Diabetes education and counselling is a lifelong, ongoing process integral to effective diabetes self-care and is an essential aspect of diabetes management. People with diabetes need appropriate general health and diabetes-specific information to enable them to manage their diabetes, problem-solve, and feel independent and in control. People require various types of information to improve their health outcomes such as preventive health care including vaccinations, and like to receive information about research and technological advances.

Education processes

Written information can supplement verbal information, provided it is in a format and language the individual understands. There are many sources of information about diabetes, including the internet, not all of which is accurate or reliable. Even if it is, it may not suit the reading ability, cultural needs, or learning style of the individual. They may also need to know how to assess the veracity of information they find in these sources.

Diabetes education can occur individually or in group sessions: each has advantages and disadvantages, depending on the teaching style and the individual's learning style. The type of information needed, and often the learning style, changes over time due to changes in disease status, cognitive ability, management changes, and increasing age. Health professionals' knowledge, competence and education style are integral to achieving congruent health professional/patient decisions. Health professionals need listening skills, the ability to develop a therapeutic relationship with the individual, and be able to identify and teach 'at teachable moments.' To do this effectively, they must be aware of their abilities and how their beliefs and attitudes affect their own behaviours and so people with diabetes.

Aims of diabetes education

The main aims of diabetes education are to assist people to

- accept their diabetes;
- develop problem-solving skills;
- integrate diabetes self-management tasks into their lifestyle; to
- achieve and maintain a balanced lifestyle and optimum metabolic control.

The following issues need to be assessed and accommodated to design empowering education encounters:

- the individual's feelings, beliefs and attitudes and his or her life goals;
- psychological status;

- spirituality, which in this case refers to self-concept, mastery and meaningfulness;
- social and environmental situation;
- education level;
- coping style;
- learning style;
- goals for the session and plans for future education sessions; and
- physical, mental, and cognitive ability to carry out self-care behaviours.

Over time, advancing age and diabetes can affect memory. Several mechanisms have been suggested for diabetes effects on memory, including cerebral damage from frequent severe hypoglycaemia, cerebrovascular disease and tissue glycosylation due to persistent hyperglycaemia. Older people (> 65 years) are at risk of dementia and cognitive decline due to vascular dementia, Alzheimer's disease, cerebral atrophy and subclinical cerebrovascular lesions (Ryan and Geckle 2000).

These conditions contribute to memory and learning problems. However, memory and learning are multifactorial and are also affected by the education process and the relationship with the educator. If present, they put the individual at risk of poor outcomes and represent a clinical challenge for health professionals and the family. Decisions about self-care ability and safety may need to be made.

Diabetes education is appropriate and essential, but knowledge alone does not necessarily result in appropriate health behaviours or self-care. Beliefs, attitudes, satisfaction and disease status are some of the factors that affect knowledge and behaviour. These factors may change over time and need to be assessed on a regular basis, for example:

- deciding what is happening at a particular time;
- what could/will change; and
- how the change could affect the individual and his or her relatives, or care needs.

An example might be the development of a diabetes complication such as retinopathy or the normal changes associated with aging.

Survival skills education

The key objectives of diabetes education for children and young people and their families are no different from that of adults diagnosed with type 1, type 2, or gestational diabetes. Diabetes education provides the knowledge, skills and tools to empower the person to self-manage. Traditional models of care for newly diagnosed children and young people are changing. There is a trend towards providing more education within an ambulatory setting rather than prolonging a hospital admission. Consensus guidelines identify that 'survival skills education' should occur in 1- to 2-hourly sessions over four to five sessions (inpatient and increasingly now as an outpatient) or within 2–3 weeks following diagnosis. Ongoing education should occur within the first 12 months of diagnosis. Education sessions should use a variety of strategies lasting 1–2 hours in duration over 8–16 sessions. Longer term, there should be at least one annual education review.

Empowerment

Empowerment models of diabetes education are based on shared governance and consideration of the whole person and their environment (Coulter 1997). Empowerment models became more common when health professionals realised that people with diabetes must be, and mostly want to be, responsible for their own care. Empowerment is based on three basic characteristics:

(1) The person with diabetes makes choices that affect his or her health care.
(2) The individual is in control of what he/she learns and the self-care practices he/she adopts.
(3) The consequences of these choices affect the person's diabetes outcomes (Anderson *et al.* 1996).

Not only are individuals taught about the disease diabetes and how to care for themselves, they are encouraged to apply the information to their personal circumstances and make decisions based on information such as their blood glucose pattern, activity level, food intake and travel. By using the information the education is reinforced and people are more likely to understand the concepts better because they have a personal meaning. Education should focus on helping the person know his or her diabetes, develop self-efficacy and self-confidence, and promote decision-making skills. Health professionals need to understand the individual's life priorities and perceived benefit and risk of diabetes and the management suggestions being offered (Fiandt 2007).

However, diabetes education and knowledge do not necessarily lead to appropriate self-care. Health professionals must focus on the psychological and social aspects of a person's life and blend counselling techniques with education strategies to encompass the complex nature of each individual and make each learning encounter relevant to his or her needs (Knight *et al.* 2006).

Many different educational programmes and a vast amount of written information are available. These include:

- Blood Glucose Awareness Training (BGAT);
- X-PERT (*www.xpert-diabetes.org.uk*);
- Dose Adjustment for Normal Eating (DAFNE) (*www.dafne.uk.com*);
- Diabetes Education and Self-Management for Ongoing and Newly Diagnosed (DESMOND) (*www.desmond-project.org.uk*);
- peer education.

However, many do not have behavioural components and not all of them address psychosocial and environment issues. Pictorial and visual aids can be very useful if an individual has language difficulties. However, a recent review of diabetes education interventions found that only 50% included behavioural components or counselling techniques (Knight *et al.* 2006). Only one-third assessed individual abilities such as self-efficacy, locus of control or abilities to undertake self-care.

CASE DISCUSSION

Mr TE

Mr TE was an inpatient and was referred to a diabetes educator
Mr TE is a 78-year-old man with type 2 diabetes who has a history of cancer and was referred because he is having trouble testing his blood glucose levels, especially obtaining enough blood.
He has:
Peripheral neuropathy
Peripheral vascular disease
Hypertension
Hyperlipidaemia.
HbA_{1c} is consistently ~7% and he takes particular care of his health.

Current medications
Xalatan eye drops (latanoprost)
Diabex (metformin)   850 mg BD
Daonil (glibenclamide)   2.5 mg if blood glucose > 10 mmol/L
Verapamil
Lipitor (atorvastatin)   dose not provided on the referral
Lactulose

He has trouble hearing.
His blood glucose lancet device is very dirty.

Diabetes educator

I would ask Mr TE's relatives to bring all his testing equipment in so I could check it and his testing technique. There may be an easier meter and fingerpricking device for him to use. I would check his vision.

It sometimes helps if the fingers are warmed by gentle massaging in a downward way from the palm to the fingertip, or in warm water before testing. Waiting for a few seconds after pricking the finger before starting to squeeze a drop of blood sometimes helps, as does pricking on the fleshy part of the side of the finger. Keeping the hand lower than the level of the heart might also help (see Box 3.1).

Endocrinologist

The presence of peripheral neuropathy suggests his control may not be as good as the HbA_{1c} suggests and careful correlation with fingerprick records is needed, and possibly fructosamine evaluation. Because of the peripheral vascular disease Mr TE needs aggressive cardiovascular risk modification and vascular specialist assessment. Targets would include BP < 120/80, LDL < 2.0, and excellent glucose control. I would not use metformin or glibenclamide in a person in this age group but prefer shorter-acting sulphonylureas such as gliclazide, which carry a lower risk of hypoglycaemia. If Mr TE has significant hand neuropathic symptoms, which impair his dexterity, nerve conduction studies to exclude additional carpal tunnel syndrome would be warranted.

CASE DISCUSSION

Mr MS

Mr MS was referred to the diabetes educator by a nurse working in general practice

Mr MS was diagnosed with type 1 diabetes 10 years ago following a 7-kg weight loss, polyuria and polydipsia. His blood glucose was 55 mmol/L at the time. He was commenced on Actrapid and Protaphane insulin BD. Six months later his blood glucose averaged ~9 mmol/L and his HbA_{1c} was 6.9%.

Eighteen months later he had lost another 4 kg, and his home blood glucose tests were all 6–8 mmol/L. However, a laboratory test showed blood glucose 16.9 mmol/L postprandially and his HbA_{1c} was 10%.

The discrepancy is still present. We have checked his testing technique, meter and strips and all seems to be in order. However, when we checked the meter memory we found only half the tests recorded in his blood glucose record book and of these many were reduced from high readings.

We are not sure how to handle this issue. I do not want to accuse him of cheating but he needs to know how important testing and accuracy are.

Please help.

Diabetes educator

It would be useful to know how old Mr MS is. The behaviours described are very common during adolescence. It would be important to explore his relationships with his family, friends and at school/work. If he is a young person, respecting his privacy and independence is important. After 10 years of diabetes he may be tired of dealing with the relentless self-care tasks and meeting the expectations of his family and health professionals (Conrad and Gitelman 2006). Worsening control might also be due to hormonal changes.

He may have been having frequent hypos when his HbA_{1c} was 6.9%. Hypos are feared and hated and many people deliberately run their blood glucose levels high to avoid hypos. His current HbA_{1c} and blood glucose has increased, which suggests his usual blood glucose is high. The weight loss is a concern and could be due to hyperglycaemia, an underlying disease process such as thyroid disease, an eating disorder, or depression/psychiatric disorder.

Early identification of the causes of any difficulty coping with diabetes is essential. The coping styles of young people with type 1 diabetes are associated with the level of metabolic control (Graue *et al.* 2004) and coping can be affected by excursions in blood glucose levels as well as illness and psychological factors. It may not be a passing phase: adverse metabolic and psychiatric outcomes occur in around one-third of young adults with diabetes (Bryden *et al.* 2003). A very careful history will help clarify the most likely cause. Alcohol consumption, illicit drug use, and stress all need to be considered and asked about with extreme care and sensitivity.

Blood glucose meters have been in use for around 30 years and have improved in accuracy and precision in that time. Laboratory (usually venous) and capillary blood cannot be directly compared. Capillary blood is approximately 10–15% higher than venous blood. I would check his meter is set for millimoles per litre rather than milligrammes per decilitre (used in the USA).

Falsifying results is a well-known multifactorial phenomenon and needs to be discussed in a non-judgmental manner.

Differences among logbooks, meter memory, and laboratory values may be an indicator of underlying stress. Language such as 'good' and 'bad' with respect to blood glucose levels is not helpful and can be interpreted by the patient as 'you are bad,' which exacerbates the problem. The discrepancy between the record and meter memory can be used as an opportunity to explore Mr MS' feelings about his diabetes and his interpersonal relationships.

I would check his insulin technique and injection sites. A more flexible insulin regimen using basal bolus regimen and insulin analogues (see Chapter 5) may give him more choice and independence. He may achieve better control and lifestyle using an insulin pump. I would refer him to an endocrinologist for careful review and possibly to a psychologist if practicable.

An overnight continuous glucose sensor monitor (CGSM) could provide useful information about the fluctuations in blood glucose levels. CGS monitoring is a useful teaching tool and could be used to provide positive feedback about what he is doing well. It is essential that trust is developed and maintained so that he is not 'lost to follow-up.' The family may also need support and advice about how to support Mr MS.

Diabetes educator 2

I would check how he is storing his test strips. They need to be in date and stored away from heat, light and moisture (in the container with the lid on/foil packages). The meter features could also be checked to ensure the date, time and other settings are correct.

I would slowly scroll through the memory results and discuss the last few with him and try to sort out together why the record book and meter memory do not match. He may not need to record in both places, which might also reduce the burden on him.

I would also check his insulin technique to ensure he is mixing correctly and giving the correct dose.

CASE DISCUSSION

> **Mr PLO**
>
> ***Mr PLO self-referred to the diabetes centre for advice***
> Can you please show me how to look after my blood glucose meter properly?
>   My GP told me it was very dirty and I should take more care with my belongings because things are not reliable otherwise.

Diabetes educator

The blood glucose meter does need to be cleaned, calibrated and control tested regularly. It is a bit like having your car serviced to make sure it runs efficiently. The outside of the meter can be wiped with a damp cloth.

I would check the meter was calibrated correctly and show Mr PLO how to check for himself using the manufacturer's instructions and ensure he has the number of the manufacturer's helpline. I would explain how to perform control testing, why it is important, and the need to check both the high and low range about once per week. Control test solutions can be expensive, and expire relatively soon after the bottle is opened, so more frequent testing may not be practical for many people. Some people may not control test at all because of the cost. When meter accuracy is clearly an issue I would offer to run control tests on Mr PLO's meter every couple of weeks for him.

I would show him how to make sure his strips are in date and stored correctly. I would observe him repeating the procedure in a return demonstration in which he explained what he was doing as he completed each step.

CASE DISCUSSION

> ***E-mailed question from a newly qualified diabetes educator***
> I have just started seeing quite a few type 2 patients in my practice.
>   Should I be asking them to test their blood glucose before or after meals?
>   What is the actual relevance of each?
>   I am getting conflicting advice from my colleagues.

Diabetes educator

Testing before meals gives different information from testing after meals. As discussed in Chapter 3, experts debate the relative value of fasting and postprandial blood glucose testing. The length of time to allow after a meal before performing the postprandial test will also affect the result. Testing soon after a meal measures the post-absorptive state, whereas testing 2–3 hours after a meal reflects glucose clearance. The postprandial state lasts up to 5 hours. Factors influencing postprandial blood glucose levels include:

- loss of first phase insulin secretion, a common feature of type 2 diabetes (see Chapter 2);
- degree of insulin resistance in muscle and adipose tissue, which may be due to obesity, medicines that induce hyperglycaemia, illness and prolonged stress;
- gastric emptying time, which is affected by diet, autonomic neuropathy and other gastrointestinal diseases; and
- unsuppressed gluconeogenesis and elevated free fatty acids, for example during illness and hyperglycaemia.

The contribution of fasting glucose to the HbA_{1c} level increases as the fasting blood glucose level increases but postprandial glucose is the major contributor to HbA_{1c} levels in the normal range. Both are useful. However, it is often easier and more practical for people to test before meals. I suggest you follow the recommendations of your national diabetes association. Most associations have a website that details such information.

CASE DISCUSSION

> ***Question from a nurse working in a medical outpatients department***
> Can you please explain exactly what HbA_{1c} is.
>   Is it always the best indication of diabetes control?

Dietitian

HbA_{1c} is a blood test taken from a vein and analysed in the laboratory to help people with diabetes and health professionals understand how well the diabetes is controlled. Several assay methods are in common use. HbA_{1c} shows the average level of glucose in the blood over the last 2–3 months. People without diabetes usually have an HbA_{1c} range of 4.0–6.3% (DCCT aligned method). A person with diabetes is considered to have excellent control if they have an $HbA_{1c} < 6.6\%$. Generally speaking, the lower the HbA_{1c}, the lower the risk of developing diabetes complications.

One way of understanding HbA_{1c} is to think about glucose sticking to red blood cells. If too much glucose remains in the blood for too long, the more it sticks to the red cells and the higher the HbA_{1c}.

Diabetes educator

I agree with most of the dietitian's comments. However, some countries aim for $HbA_{1c} < 7\%$. In addition, venous samples may not be used if a DCA analyser is available. This enables HbA_{1c} to be performed on a fingerprick blood sample during the consultation, which enables the information to be used proactively during the consultation to make timely adjustments to the management regimen and as an education tool.

While HbA_{1c} is the best indication of overall blood glucose control, it can be altered by several factors and needs to be considered in the context of the individual (see Chapter 3).

HbA_{1c} corresponds with circulating blood glucose representing approximately 50% in the first month and 25% in the second and third months.

The HbA_{1c} level can be lower when the survival time of red blood cells is reduced; for example, due to anaemia and abnormal haemoglobin types such as fetal haemoglobin or sickle cells, recent blood loss, blood transfusions, and frequent hypoglycaemia. Carbamylated haemoglobin, which occurs in uraemic syndromes, can lead to higher levels.

HbA_{1c} is usually tested at least 3 months apart but can be done sooner to gauge the effect of a treatment modification. A change of 0.5% reflects a true change.

CASE DISCUSSION

Mrs TKAT

Mrs TKAT telephoned the diabetes educator to ask about her blurred vision, which got worse after she started insulin

---

Diabetes educator

It is not uncommon for people to experience visual changes after their blood glucose control improves. It is usually a temporary problem, which corrects without treatment and which is not sight-threatening. When the blood glucose is high, glucose readily enters the lens of the eye and can cause visual changes due to the effects on the lens. Many people actually visit an 'eye doctor' or optometrist to have their vision checked and the diagnosis of diabetes is made at that time. This is different from retinal changes, which occur in the longer term and are sight-threatening.

As the blood glucose control improves with treatment, the excess glucose in the lens begins to leach out, which again causes visual changes. The process usually lasts 6–8 weeks. Any sudden visual changes or vision problems persisting longer than 6 weeks should be assessed. All people with type 2 diabetes should have an eye check at diagnosis and then at regular intervals. People with type 1 should have regular screening from about age 10.

References

Anderson R, Funnel M, Arnold M (1996) Using the empowerment approach to help patients change behaviour. In: Anderson B, Rubin R (eds) *Practical Psychology for Clinicians*. American Diabetes Association, Alexandria, pp 163–172.

Bryden K, Dunger D, Mayou R *et al.* (2003) Poor prognosis of young adults with type 1 diabetes. *Diabetes Care* 26: 1052–1057.

Conrad S, Gitelman S (2006) If the numbers don't fit . . . discrepancies between glucose meter readings and hemoglobin A1c reveal stress of living with diabetes. *Clinical Diabetes* 24: 45–47.

Coulter A (1997) Partnerships with patients: the pros and cons of shared clinical decision making. *Journal of Health Service Policy* 2: 112–121.

Fiandt K (2007) The chronic care model: description and application for practice. *Topics in Advanced Practice Nursing eJournal* 6(4): posted 5 January 2007.

Graue M, Wentzel-Larsen T, Bru E *et al.* (2004) The coping styles of adolescents with type 1 diabetes are associated with degree of metabolic control. *Diabetes Care* 27: 1313–1317.

Knight KM, Dornan T, Bundy C (2006) The diabetes educator: trying hard but must concentrate more on behaviour. *Diabetic Medicine* 23: 485–501.

Ryan C, Geckle M (2000) Why is memory and learning dysfunction in type 2 diabetes limited to older adults? *Diabetes Metabolism and Research Reviews* 16(5): 308–315.

Tibbetts C (2006) Diabetes self-management education: a saga of angels and demons. *Diabetes Spectrum* 19: 54–57.

Recommended reading

Cox D, Gonder-Frederick L (1992) Major developments in behavioural diabetes research. *Journal of Consulting Clinical Psychologists* 60: 628–638.

International Diabetes Federation Consultative Section on Diabetes Education (IDF–DECS) (1997) *International Consensus Standards of Practice for Diabetes Education*. IDF, Brussels.

Chapter 10

Gestational diabetes

Key points

- Gestational diabetes occurs in 2–9% of all pregnancies.
- Women who develop gestational diabetes are at increased risk of developing type 2 diabetes.
- If diet and exercise do not control blood glucose, insulin will be required.

Introduction

Gestational diabetes mellitus (GDM) occurs in 2–9% of all pregnancies (Hoffman *et al.* 1998). Evidence suggests that the use of insulin in treating high blood glucose levels in GDM reduces serious perinatal morbidity (Crowther *et al.* 2005). Pregnancy is an exciting time in a woman's life. However, once the diagnosis of GDM is made, the pregnancy will be managed at a more intensive level of care. GDM is managed using diet and exercise but one in six women (or 16%) with GDM requires insulin. The care is usually transferred from the general practitioner to a multidisciplinary team that consists of an obstetrician, endocrinologist, diabetes educator and dietitian.

Experts face the dilemma of managing GDM on a regular basis in diabetes centres. The potential need for insulin should be addressed promptly to improve fetal and maternal outcomes, and reduce maternal anxiety about the blood glucose levels and the impact they could have on the developing fetus, and the fear of the prospect of giving insulin injections.

Managing gestational diabetes

The diabetes educator will teach the woman with GDM how to closely monitor her blood glucose levels (HBGM) and will usually lend her a blood glucose meter until after the delivery. Ideally, women should test their blood glucose four times a day, usually before breakfast and 2 hours after each meal. The dietitian's role is to focus on providing culturally relevant, healthy eating advice in pregnancy and help plan a sensible exercise routine within the constraints of advancing pregnancy. If, after a week on diet and exercise, HBGM reveals that the target levels of < 5.5 mmol/L fasting and/or < 7.0 mmol/L 2 hours postprandial (Hoffman *et al.* 1998) are not achieved, insulin may be required.

Some centres use lower HBGM targets, for example < 5 mmol/L fasting and < 6.5 mmol/L 2 hours postprandial. Between 10% and 25% of women with GDM require insulin during pregnancy (Australian Diabetes in Pregnancy Society) so it is advisable to approach the initial education with a view that insulin may be required if HBGM targets are not achieved despite every endeavour. It is very important to reassure the woman that she is not to blame and to explain why the blood glucose goes high, even if it was explained earlier. As the pregnancy advances, the production of the pregnancy hormones, oestrogen, progesterone, cortisol and human placental lactogen, collectively result in insulin resistance, and endogenous insulin may not be adequate to keep blood glucose levels within the normal range. The results of the recent Australian Carbohydrate Intolerance Study suggest that insulin treatment improves outcome in GDM (Crowther *et al.* 2005).

Women often become concerned when insulin treatment is recommended. They often feel guilty as well as being concerned about the risk to their babies. They often ask themselves (and their health professionals) why they 'failed' and try to 'fix' the problem by avoiding carbohydrates. This is contraindicated because, when fat is metabolised as an alternative energy source, ketones are produced. Ketonemia may have an adverse effect on the neurological development of the fetus. Recent research also suggests that children of mothers with diabetes who had fluctuating blood glucose levels during pregnancy perform worse than controls on some memory tests at one year and three and a half years ($n = 20$) (DeBoer *et al.* 2007). The researchers attribute the effects to inadequate oxygen and iron levels reaching the fetal hippocampus. Iron is conserved in the fetus to form haemoglobin, which results in lower levels of iron reaching the brain. The brain requires a large amount of iron, which is involved in laying down neurone in the hippocampus.

There is also the possibility that the woman only records HBGM results within the target ranges. Meters have the capacity to store up to 450 individual blood glucose results, which can be downloaded onto a computer. Downloading the HBGM results provides important information and can be used as a teaching tool.

Commencing insulin

An important consideration is whether commencing insulin will improve outcomes. The emotional impact of the diagnosis on both the mother and the father should not be underestimated. Any fears or anxieties should be addressed promptly through discussion with the couple, allowing adequate time for questions. If counselling services are necessary, prompt referral to a psychologist is recommended. The mother is expected to self-inject between one and four times a day, perform HBGM more frequently, and is at risk of developing hypoglycaemia. The timing or mode of delivery could be changed due to 'nervousness' by the obstetrician as the woman nears term. Obstetric and diabetes follow-up appointments need to be more frequent, generally weekly from 34 weeks onwards when the woman is on insulin.

Generally, insulin is only required during the pregnancy and blood glucose levels rapidly return to normal after the delivery. Health professionals must remind women they have 30% to 50% risk of developing type 2 diabetes in 5–20 years and the lifestyle changes they made during pregnancy are needed for life (Drucquer and McNally 1998; Cohen 2000; Knowler *et al.* (Diabetes Prevention Group) 2002). The diagnosis of GDM is a wake-up call for many women and a chance to adopt a healthy lifestyle to reduce the risk of diabetes mellitus in the future. Women with GDM should have an oral glucose tolerance test (OGTT) every 1–2 years for life. Follow-up is usually organised by the general practitioner. Maintenance of healthy body weight, regular exercise, and healthy lifestyle choices reduce the risk of type 2 diabetes in the future.

CASE DISCUSSION

Mrs ORA

Mrs ORA was referred to a diabetes educator when she developed diabetes at 29.5 weeks' gestation
Mrs ORA is a 30-year-old primigravida and is 29.5 weeks pregnant.

She was referred to the diabetes educator from the antenatal clinic because her oral glucose tolerance test showed her BG was elevated at 8.7 mmol/L 2 hours after a 75-g glucose load.

Diabetes educator

The key educational issues for Mrs ORA are:

- Understand the importance of home blood glucose monitoring in gestational diabetes.
- Decide when to start insulin in gestational diabetes mellitus.
- Allay the woman's fears about the impact of insulin treatment during the pregnancy.
- Enable self-management of injections.
- Prepare the woman for delivery and possibility of diabetes in the future.

The diabetes educator arranged for Mrs ORA to be reviewed by the diabetes team. At the initial consultation it was important to reassure her and gain her trust. Mrs ORA was taught to perform HBGM using a loan hospital blood glucose meter and was given dietary advice by the dietitian. Exercise within the limitations of advancing pregnancy was also encouraged. In Australia, women with GDM are registered through the National Diabetes Services Scheme (NDSS) for the duration of the pregnancy, enabling them to get blood glucose test strips at heavily subsidised prices. On review 1 week later, despite following the dietary advice and walking 20 minutes a day, Mrs ORA's blood glucose levels remained above the target goals.

The results in Table 10.1 clearly indicate the need for insulin, because more than 50% of the readings are > 5.5 mmol/L fasting or > 7.0 mmol/L 2 hours after meals. The Australian Diabetes in Pregnancy Society suggest that insulin should be considered if BGLs exceed the targets on two or more occasions in a 1- to 2-week period, particularly in the presence of macrosomia as determined by ultrasound. The insulin regimen should be tailored to address the times when hyperglycaemia occurs. The table shows Mrs ORA has hyperglycaemia before breakfast and 2 hours after meals. She was prescribed a basal bolus regimen of a short-acting analogue with meals, and intermediate-acting insulin at bedtime.

While there are no adequate well controlled studies in pregnant women, the shorter-acting insulin analogues, for example Humalog and NovoRapid, and the longer-acting insulin analogues, such as Lantus and Levemir, are preferred by some endocrinologists. This option is one that would be preferred if the benefits of improved glycaemic control or well-being of the mother (decreased hypoglycaemia, especially nocturnal events and anxiety) outweigh any possible risk of harm to the developing fetus. Mrs ORA was asked to perform HBGM before and after meals to ascertain whether glycaemic targets were being met.

Table 10.1 Mrs ORA's home blood glucose monitoring results (mmol/L).

	Breakfast Before	After	Lunch Before	After	Dinner Before	After
Monday	4.7	8.1	8.4		7.2	
Tuesday	4.5	7.0	7.1			
Wednesday	5.1				6.9	
Thursday	7.2	8.5			7.6	
Friday	6.8		7.0			
Saturday	8.1	9.1				
Sunday	7.8		6.5		8.0	
Monday	6.9	7.3	6.9			
Tuesday	6.8	6.9	7.0		6.8	
Wednesday	7.3	7.1				

Time of introducing insulin is crucial to prevent fetal macrosomia. Often, only around 10–12 weeks remain before delivery, leaving only a small window of opportunity to correct the blood glucose levels. Regular review and dose titration is necessary to achieve targets without causing hypoglycemia.

A lot of women ask 'why can't I have tablets?' Unfortunately, oral hypoglycaemic agents (OHAs) are not approved for use in GDM. Further research is needed to assess the long-term risks of fetal exposure to OHAs because of their possible teratogenic effect. Some endocrinologists do use metformin to reduce insulin resistance (Simmons *et al.* 2004), for example in the presence of polycystic ovary syndrome and type 2 diabetes, because the potential benefits outweigh the potential for harm to the fetus. Currently there are insufficient data to support using metformin in lieu of insulin in GDM.

Fetal monitoring is also increased depending on the individual woman. Weekly to twice-weekly cardiotocograph is performed from 32 weeks and ultrasound at 32 weeks to assess for fetal growth abnormalities and polyhydramnios. Repeat ultrasounds may be needed if there is any doubt about the diagnosis.

Education

In the main, women with GDM are extremely motivated and proactive in their management because their main concern is the well-being of their babies. However, they often express concern about having to give themselves an injection. Once the technique is demonstrated and they experience the first injection they realise the needle is less painful than the fingerprick. They often comment afterwards 'the injection was not that bad.' Usually women with GDM are taught to use a disposable insulin delivery device such as a FlexPen or a cartridge pen. Syringes are rarely used. Disposal of used sharps is important and initially the woman is supplied with a disposable container until she is able to acquire one from her local council. If this is not possible a solid plastic bottle with a screw top can be used as an alternative. Disposal of sharps in household garbage is discouraged. Advice should be sought from the local council about disposal regulations.

In the event of needle phobia, the PenMate, a device designed for people who dislike needles, can be used. It has an auto self-inject mechanism that slips over the NovoPen and hides the needle from view when injecting.

Reinforcing rotating injection sites, using a new needle every time, and gentle insertion enable most women to confidently manage their GDM well. Occasionally, family may be required to assist. When discussing the need for insulin, asking the woman and her family whether they have any questions or fears helps ascertain whether there are likely to be any issues such as needle phobia or failure to follow advice as recommended. Insulin stabilisation is best achieved on an ambulatory basis with close communication among the woman, the diabetes educator and endocrinologist.

The endocrinologist decides on a delivery date, usually around 37 weeks. The plan depends on the timing of delivery and becomes obsolete if the woman goes into spontaneous labour. In this situation, the woman should contact the diabetes service regarding her insulin therapy or go directly to the delivery suite and her insulin requirements and blood glucose levels will be reassessed. However, insulin is usually not required in active labour. If the blood glucose is > 7.0 mmol/L the doctor may order a dose of rapid-acting insulin. The pre-delivery plan needs to be recorded in the medical history or a letter that includes insulin instructions that the woman takes to the hospital with her. The labour ward should be aware of the insulin plan and who to contact for advice about blood glucose levels. The diabetes educator can also assist the midwives to interpret the blood glucose pattern while the woman is in labour. Usually BGM is performed 2-hourly during labour.

Insulin is not given postpartum. Occasionally it takes 24–48 hours for the blood glucose levels to return to normal. Hyperglycaemia in a normal postpartum may be directly linked to a change in dietary habits. After having spent the past few weeks being very careful, the woman may be tempted to splurge on treats initially.

Accepting that the birth is a time of celebration, the diabetes educator can gently remind the woman that these treats should always remain just that – treats.

CASE DISCUSSION

> **Mrs BY**
>
> ***Mrs BY self-referred to the diabetes educator for advice***
> I have had type I diabetes forever.
>   How frequently should newborn babies of mothers with diabetes have their blood glucose tested after birth?

Diabetes educator

The Australian Diabetes in Pregnancy Society recommends that babies have their blood tested 1 hour after delivery and before the first four feeds for the first 24 hours. It is common for the baby's blood glucose to drop on the fourth day after delivery. Hypoglycaemia in newborn babies can occur for a number of reasons such as breathing difficulties, feeding difficulties because the baby is sleepy, has difficulty attaching to the breast, or the milk has not come in sufficiently.

CASE DISCUSSION

> **Mrs SMS**
>
> ***Mrs SMS self-referred to a diabetes educator when she was diagnosed with GDM***
> I am very worried that I might have to inject insulin in case it damages my baby.

Diabetes educator

I would recognise her concern for her baby and ask what her specific concerns were so they could be addressed. Once her concerns were addressed I would explain to her that approximately one in six women with gestational diabetes need insulin to keep the blood glucose in the normal range. I would explain that high blood glucose represents far more risk to the baby (and to her) than insulin injections. I would show her the areas of the body where insulin can be injected – abdomen, thigh and upper arm – and explain the advantages and disadvantages of each area, but indicate the abdomen is preferred because insulin absorption is more predictable when injected into the abdomen.

Women worry that the needle might prick the baby. This is unlikely to happen because the needle is very short and only penetrates into the subcutaneous layers rather than through the muscle and uterine wall. I would draw a picture to explain how well protected the baby is in the uterus and where the needle penetrates to. I would explain that insulin is very safe and is almost identical to the insulin produced naturally by the body and there is no risk to the baby from the insulin.

References

Cohen M (2000) *Diabetes: A Handbook of Management for Health Professionals*, 7th edn. Servier Laboratories (Australia) Pty Ltd, Melbourne.

Crowther CA, Hiller J, Moss J *et al.* (2005) Effect of treatment of gestational diabetes mellitus on pregnancy outcomes. *New England Journal of Medicine* 352(24): 2477–2486.

DeBoer T, Wewerka S, Bauer PJ *et al.* (2005) Explicit memory performance in infants of diabetic mothers at 1 year of age. *Developmental Medicine and Child Neurology* 47(8): 525–531.

Drucquer M, McNally P (1998) *Diabetes Management, Step by Step*. Blackwell Science, London.

Hoffman L, Nolan C, Wilson J *et al.* (1998): Gestational diabetes mellitus – management guidelines: the Australian Diabetes in Pregnancy Society. *Medical Journal of Australia* 169: 93–97.

Knowler WC, Barrett-Connor E, Fowler SE *et al.* (Diabetes Prevention Program Research Group) (2002) Reduction in the incidence of type 2 diabetes with lifestyle intervention or metformin. *New England Journal of Medicine* 346: 393–403.

Simmons D, Walters B, Rowan A *et al.* (2004) Metformin therapy and diabetes in pregnancy. *Medical Journal of Australia* 180(9): 462–464.

Chapter 11

Complementary and alternative therapies

<table>
<tr><td>

Key points

- Health professionals must be non-judgmental about people's decision to use complementary therapies.
- People with diabetes frequently use complementary therapies for a variety of reasons not only to reduce blood glucose.
- Health professionals should ask about complementary therapy use.
- Complementary therapies should be used within a quality use of medicines framework.
- Not all complementary therapies are 'medicines'.

</td></tr>
</table>

Introduction

The World Health Organization (WHO) Traditional Medicine Strategy 2002–2005 described the role, challenges, and opportunities for traditional medicine in health care and recognised the vital importance of traditional medicines to the care of many people with diabetes in countries such as Africa (WHO 2002). The WHO works collaboratively with other organisations such as the United Nations and global and professional organisations including in the field of complementary health care. Many terms such as 'alternative,' 'complementary,' 'unconventional,' 'traditional,' 'natural,''unproven' and 'unscientific' are used to describe complementary and alternative medicine (CAM). Most of these terms are judgmental and prejudiced and many countries have adopted CAM (Vincent and Furnham 1997).

CAM is receiving increasing attention in the media and by the general public and health professionals. Over 50% of the world's overall population and between 25 and 30% of people with diabetes use CAM. Recently, Egede *et al.* (2002) showed that people with diabetes in the US are 1.6 times more likely to use CAM than non-diabetics. Many health professionals are beginning to incorporate CAM into their practice or refer selected patients to CAM practitioners. Conventional practitioners need to understand that CAM encompasses many therapies besides herbal medicines and people with diabetes use CAM for many reasons, not only to control blood glucose. It helps if health professionals understand CAM philosophy and the benefits as well as the risks associated with CAM use for people with diabetes.

Profile of CAM users

Over 50% of the population in most countries use some type of CAM. The percentage is higher (> 80%) in countries such as Africa where it is an essential part of health care (WHO 2002). However, the decision to use CAM is complex and multifactorial. CAM users are often:

- well educated;
- financially well off;
- women;
- people with chronic diseases including diabetes, heart disease, and chronic airways disease;
- those who are committed to the environment;
- people who experience a traumatic psychological/physical event;
- people interested in self-care who choose to be involved in their health care, which is essential for effective diabetes self-care and health outcomes (Lloyd *et al.* 1993). These findings appear to be independent of health systems and culture (Kumar *et al.* 2006);
- people who have had previous experience with CAM and the advice of significant others.

Most CAM use is self-initiated, in which case it may be used without a comprehensive health assessment, appropriate diagnosis, or adequate monitoring. Importantly, self-diagnosis and self-treatment can delay appropriate conventional or CAM treatment and/or result in adverse events such as herb-medicine interactions. Many CAM users do not inform their conventional carers about their CAM use or CAM providers about their conventional management, which increases the risk of adverse events. The individual may not deliberately withhold information. CAM users report they worry about being ridiculed or believe the doctor or diabetes educator would not be interested.

Reasons for using CAM

Commonly used CAM includes nutritional therapies and supplements, herbal medicines from a range of herbal traditions, naturopathy, massage, meditation and spiritual therapies (see Table 11.1 and Boxes 11.1 and 11.2). CAM is frequently used to maintain health, prevent minor self-limiting conditions, manage stress, and control symptoms such as pain. Empowering the individual to be self-caring and problem-solving is integral to the healing philosophies of most CAM paradigms, and is integral to effective diabetes management. In the CAM context, 'healing' refers to restoring balance, not curing disease. Significantly, the individual's specific circumstances are considered when developing a healing programme (mind, body, spirit, and the social and cultural environment) and illness is viewed as an opportunity to make positive changes to achieve life goals.

Box 11.1 Commonly used glucose-lowering herbs

These herbs are predominantly used to treat type 2 diabetes. Many are usual dietary components in some cultures. They can have additive effects with conventional glucose-lowering agents, and their exact mechanism of action is unknown, but the following effects have been proposed:

    * induces insulin secretion and/or has insulin-like action on receptors;

    † increases insulin sensitivity and reduces insulin resistance;

    ‡ reduces carbohydrate absorption and lowers postprandial blood glucose level;

    § lipid-lowering.

- *Allium sativum*
- *Langerstroemia speciosa* bamba (glucosol)*†
- *Coccinia indica* (leaves)
- *Cassia cinnamomum* (Chinese)†
- *Panax quinquefolius* (American)†
- *Panax ginseng* (Asia)†
- Ginseng (unspecified species)
- *Gymnema sylvestre* (Gumar)*
- *Momordica charantica** (polypeptide-p, a plant insulin with similar action to bovine insulin)
- *Momordica charantia* (Karolla)
- *Ocimum* (basil, unspecified species)
- *Ocimum sanctum* (holy basil)
- *Opuntia streptacantha* lemaire and nopal (prickly pear)†‡
- *Trigonella goenum* graceum (fenugreek)†‡
- *Silybum marianum* (milk thistle)
- *Stevia rebaudiana*, which is also a non-calorie sweetener

Other glucose-lowering herbs include:

- *Pterocarpus marsupium* (India)
- *Camellia sinensis* (green tea)
- *Acacia catechu* (Burma)
- *Vaccinium myrtilus* (bilberry, Europe)
- *Atriplex halimus* (saltbush, Israel)
- *Aloe vera* (Arabian peninsula)

Metformin is derived from *Galega officinalis* (goat's rue).

Box 11.2 CAM lipid-lowering agents grouped according to their proposed mechanism of action

They have the potential to interact with conventional medicines that have similar mechanisms of action.

They inhibit cholesterol absorption by slowing gastric emptying and reduce postprandial lipid and glucose absorption.

- *Hordeum vulgare* (barley)
- *Plantago ovata* (blond psyllium)
- *Avena sativa* (oat bran)
- Chitosan
- Sitostanols
- Guar gum

Natural HMG-CoA reductase inhibitors

- *Cyanara cardunculus* (artichoke)
- *Allium sativum* (garlic)
- Policosanol, which is derived from sugar cane and increases HDL
- *Monascus purpureus* (red rice)
- Niacin

Fish oil fatty acids

- DHA
- EPA

Others
Commiphora wightii (guggul)

Herbal and nutritional therapies

People with diabetes try various diets such as the ABO blood type, Pritikin and Ornish, and the Atkins diet, and nutritional supplements such as vitamins E, B group and C as well as mineral supplements (Di

Table 11.1 Commonly used complementary therapies presented in groups or categories, with examples of some specific modalities within each group.

Complementary therapy group	Example therapies
Ayurveda (Indian traditional healing system): concerned with balancing doshas or subtle energies in the body	Herbal medicines Surgery Diet Exercise such as yoga Massage with or without essential oils Mediation
Chinese medicine: concerned with maintaining/restoring balance and harmony (Yin Yang)	Herbal medicines Acupuncture Exercise such as Tai Chi and Qi Gong Cupping Moxibustion Diet
Bodywork	Massage Reflexology
Essential oils (aromatherapy)	Vapourisation Massage Internal use in some countries
Chiropractic and manipulative therapies	Osteopathy
Naturopathy	Diet Exercise Herbal medicines
Phytomedicine, often called herbal medicine	Herbal medical traditions: – Chinese – Indian – American Indian – Asian – Australian Aboriginal – European – Tibetan Nutrition and supplements
Energetic therapies	Therapeutic touch Holistic touch Qi Gong Homeopathy Reiki Electromagnetic fields and magnet therapies Flower essences
Mind–body therapies	Meditation Music Hypnosis and self-hypnosis Self-help Visualisation Biofeedback techniques Prayer Spiritual healing
Pet therapy	Riding for the disabled Therapy animals, especially dogs

Vincenzo 2006; see Box 11.1). Some of the diets are similar to those recommended by conventional practitioners, others are deficient in carbohydrate and fibre. The value of supplementation when there is not a clear deficiency is widely debated. Oxidative stress and the consequent free radical production is implicated in the development of many diseases including diabetes and vascular disease and diets rich in antioxidant foods are associated with lower risk (McKay 2007). However, Bjelakovic *et al.* (2007) suggest free radicals could be markers of disease rather than the cause of disease. People should be advised to improve their dietary intake of antioxidant foods and not exceed recommended safe levels if they choose to supplement. Smokers and healthy older women are the most likely to benefit (Liu *et al.* 2006).

A number of herbal medicines (often complex herbal formulas) are used to manage blood glucose (Box 11.1) and lipid levels (Box 11.2), and control blood pressure, as well as for concomitant diseases and intercurrent illnesses, for example B group vitamins and alpha-lipoic acid in painful neuropathy. It is important to check assumptions about why people use CAM. Safety and efficacy of most herbal therapies is based on a long history of traditional use, sometimes confirmed in randomised trials.

Manufacturing practices lead to adulteration, contamination and variation in the ingredients and proportions (dose-to-dose variations) in herbal medicines in some countries and represent a significant health risk. In addition, herbs are sometimes incorrectly identified. It is vital that the full botanical name is used rather than common names. Labels can be misleading and do not contain sufficient information to enable safe informed use. Herbal medicines can interact with conventional medicines and other herbs. Such interactions can be harmful: some are beneficial.

In Australia, herbal medicines are regulated by the Therapeutic Goods Association (TGA) and carry an Aust L sign on the label, which signifies the medicine is considered safe but does not guarantee efficacy: or an Aust R label, which indicates the medicine has undergone rigorous testing and is safe and effective. Manufacturers must conform to good manufacturing practices, codes and regulations.

More than 700 herbs and some 1200 herbal constituents have demonstrated hypoglycaemic properties. Commonly used glucose-lowering herbs are shown in Box 11.1. Herbal therapies are rarely used to manage blood glucose in type 1 diabetes in developed countries but they may be the only treatment available in some countries (WHO 2002). Chromium has been shown to reduce insulin resistance and is also used to manage insulin resistance due to polycystic ovarian syndrome (Natural Medicines Comprehensive Database 2006). Lipid-lowering herbs and supplements are also widely used (see Box 11.2).

Complementary and conventional medicine interactions

Safety is a key aspect of medicine management but safety is a complex issue (Braun 2006). A number of diabetes-specific adverse events from using CAM have been reported. These include:

- infection, trauma and burns to neuropathic legs following cupping and moxibustion;
- bruising following an aromatherapy massage in a patient taking warfarin. The pressure of the massage rather than the essential oils used in the massage may have caused the bruising;
- hypoglycaemia from combining Chinese or Ayurveda herbal medicines and conventional hypoglycaemic medicines;
- hyperglycaemia, secondary to consuming iodine-containing herbs that caused thyroid dysfunction;
- toxicity from contaminated and adulterated herbal products and incorrectly labelled herbs in herbal products;
- stopping insulin in type 1 diabetes leading to ketoacidosis;
- chromium supplements in the presence of renal disease;
- reduced absorption of the herbal medicine in the presence of gastric stasis and taking with some foods. Nutrient absorption such as calcium, iron, and vitamin B12 can also be affected. The individual should be advised to take the medicine 1 hour before or 4 hours after food.

Many herbal–conventional medicine interactions are theoretical and speculative or based on single case reports. Some indications that an interaction is possible, when they are most likely to occur and what to do in these circumstances are shown in Table 11.2. The following potential interactions should be considered in people with diabetes who use CAM and conventional medications together:

- Hypoglycaemia is possible if glucose-lowering herbal and conventional medicines are combined.
- Hawthorn is used to control blood pressure because of its ACE inhibitor effects. Hawthorn may have additive effects when used with antihypertensive agents and cause hypotension. Alternatively

it may enable a lower dose of conventional medicines to be used.

- Potassium supplements can increase the risk of hyperkalaemia when combined with angiotensin converting enzyme (ACE-I) and potassium-sparing diuretics.
- Calcium supplements may reduce the hypotensive activity of some calcium channel blockers.
- Glucosamine is commonly used to reduce joint inflammation and is recommended by many 'arthritis associations'. Theoretically, glucosamine can cause hyperglycaemia, but clinical trials indicate this is not the case (Anderson 2005). Glucosamine sulphate might cause allergy in individuals sensitive to shellfish.
- St. John's Wort is used to treat mild to moderate depression. Because it is associated with a number of interactions especially with anticoagulants it should be used with caution, regularly monitored, and the dose reduced slowly. St. John's Wort should be stopped for 2–3 days before surgery. It may reduce blood levels of simvastatin.
- Kelp, iodine supplements, and spirulina with kelp may alter thyroid function and affect blood glucose levels.
- Garlic, Gingko biloba, St. John's Wort, soy protein, fenugreek, and vitamin E in large doses may cause bleeding if they are used with anticoagulant medications. Many foods contain flavonoids, which interfere with platelet activity, for example grapefruit, chocolate, wine, and cocoa (Faraday 2006).
- Grapefruit juice and bitter orange, but not sweet orange, interact with simvastatin, atorvastatin, and cyclosporin.
- Co-enzyme Q10 may precipitate hypoglycaemia if it is used with oral hypoglycaemic agents. It may enable lower doses of statins to be used, since it has been shown to reduce LDL and cholesterol oxidation.
- Cranberry juice is often used prophylactically to reduce the risk of urinary tract infections. Preliminary data suggest it may increase the international normalised ratio (INR) in patients on warfarin (Grant 2004) but the evidence is conflicting. A beneficial interaction is that it increases absorption of vitamin B12 when used with proton pump inhibitors (Saltzman *et al.* 1994).

Table 11.2 Indicators of herb/conventional medicine interactions, situations likely to result in an interaction, and the process to follow if an interaction occurs or is suspected.

Situations likely to result in an adverse interaction	Indicators of a herb/ conventional medicine interaction	Process to follow
Medicines have a narrow therapeutic index, e.g. warfarin, digoxin	When a condition that has been stable suddenly improves or worsens	Ask the patient about the conventional, CAM, and non-prescription medicines he/she is taking in an objective, non-judgmental manner. Ideally this occurs routinely as part of medication monitoring
The medical condition is serious with significant metabolic disturbance	When a new herbal or conventional medicine is added to the regimen	Stop the herb or conventional medicine depending on the patient's condition and indications for the medicines concerned
		Monitor the effects and adjust doses as indicated
		Collect a sample of the herbal medicine if possible so it can be analysed. Sometimes contaminants rather than the herb cause adverse events
		Complete an adverse medicine reaction form and send it to the relevant monitoring authority
		Document the event and processes followed in the person's medical record
		Record the fact that an adverse medicine-related event occurred if the interaction is substantiated
When the herb and conventional medicine are both metabolised by the same cytochrome P450 liver enzyme system or rely on the same transport system	When the herb or conventional medicines that were effective become less effective	
Presence of medical conditions such as cardiac, renal and liver disease, which affect herb and conventional medicine pharmacodynamics and pharmacokinetics	When the herb or conventional medicine dose needs to be increased to maintain its effect	
When the chemical composition of a herb includes constituents such as alkaloids and cardiac glycosides	When a complication or comorbidity develops	
When the herb affects blood glucose		
When the herb affects platelet function		

CASE DISCUSSION

> **Mr YM**
>
> ***Mr YM was referred by his GP***
> Mr YM had a recent diagnosis of type 2 diabetes. He was referred to the diabetes educator and dietitian. When he was reviewed by the GP he stated:
> 'It is now 3 years since I was diagnosed with diabetes. At first I was very upset and then I read lots of books about it and joined Diabetes Australia.
> The dietitian turned my eating habits upside down. The diabetes educator demanded too much attention and time during the day, as if I had nothing else to do or think of. I also consulted herbalists and talked to other people with diabetes.
> My diabetes is now so much under control without prescribed medicine that I only really think about it in the mornings. I wash my hands with soap and use a paper towel to wipe and prick my finger. Then I have a drink, take chromium and brindleberry tablets and have a good breakfast of wholemeal bread and two cooked eggs, or sardines or porridge with fruit salad, or leftover mixed vegetables. This keeps me going during the day and stops the hunger pangs. I put low calorie cream cheese on bread or nothing.
> I test my BGL 2 hours after every new food item and keep a diary. This helps me to know what food affects my diabetes.'

Dietitian

I would need to obtain clinical results such as HbA_{1c}, blood pressure readings, lipid profile, albumin:creatinine ratio, BMI and waist circumference. I would refer Mr YM for a foot assessment and retinal eye screening. I would also need to clarify whether he was originally prescribed oral hypoglycaemic medications that he has stopped taking in preference for alternative therapies.

I would ask Mr YM the following questions:

- What do you believe is the benefit of taking chromium and brindleberry tablets?
- What do you mean by 'the dietitian turned my eating habits upside down'?
- Did you find the advice beneficial? If not, why?
- What is your current dietary intake?
- How have you changed your diet since you were diagnosed with type 2 diabetes?
- Are you happy with your present diet and body weight?
- Would it be more convenient for you to attend structured/self-management education during the evening or work through a CDROM/DVD at home?

I would also determine whether he had been taught the correct technique for blood glucose self-monitoring.

Depending on his responses to these questions and his degree of willingness I would:

- Refer him for structured/self-management education where he is able to develop the knowledge and skills to perform a dietary self-assessment. If he is able to analyse his own diet he will be able to make an informed decision regarding whether his diet is nutritionally balanced and benefiting his diabetes control.
- Inform him that there is very little evidence that chromium assists in the management of blood glucose control. Although some studies have shown a benefit, these were performed a long time ago in people from Asia. A recent study concluded there is no benefit in taking chromium supplements for diabetes if people are consuming a well-balanced diet (Kleefstra *et al.* 2006). I would inform Mr YM that it is difficult to find any evidence for supplementing the diet with brindleberry tablets; although these supplements are unlikely to do any harm, they are likely to be expensive.

Diabetes educator

Mr YM's comments suggested he initially found it difficult to come to terms with the diagnosis of diabetes and found the required self-care and advice burdensome. In the 3 years since the diagnosis he appears to have come to terms with his diabetes and taken some proactive steps to manage the disease. In addition, he has declared his interest in CAM to his GP and openly discussed the CAM he uses. It would be important to determine whether he is using OHA or whether he is controlling his blood glucose using diet and CAM. It would also be useful to determine his blood glucose pattern, lipid levels, and HbA_{1c}.

Chromium is essential to normal carbohydrate metabolism and enhances insulin sensitivity and glucose transport into cells. In addition, it may reduce total cholesterol, LDL, and triglycerides (Preuss *et al.* 2000) and has positive effects on bone density (McCarty 1995). Trivalent chromium (chromium picolinate) is the form most commonly used. While research into the glucose-lowering effects of chromium is contradictory, positive effects appear to be more likely in people with glucose intolerance like Mr YM, but the effects are difficult to predict (Gunton *et al.* 2005). Therefore, Mr YM's blood glucose tests and laboratory results will be an important guide to the benefits of chromium. If he were taking OHAs as well, I would advise him about the possibility of hypoglycaemia. If he is on lipid-lowering medicines, his medicine dose requirements should be monitored.

Brindleberry (*Garcinia cambogia*) is often used as a weight loss herb, which induces a feeling of fullness, and may increase serotonin levels and reduce appetite. A major compound, hydroxycitric acid (HCA), which is related to citric acid in citrus fruits, blocks the conversion of sugar to starch and starch to fat. The usual dose is 750–2000 mg/day. Brindleberry is an ingredient in several weight loss formulas and is often combined with glucose-lowering herbs such as gymnema. Brindleberry can interact with conventional medicines and is contraindicated in pregnancy, but there is limited evidence about the risks and benefits (Egger *et al.* 1999).

CASE DISCUSSION

Mr AD

Mr AD self-referred to the diabetes educator for advice
Mr AD is 20 and was diagnosed with type 1 diabetes 3 months previously after moving from the country to the city to commence university studies.

He was commenced on a basal bolus regime: NovoRapid 6 units before each meal and Protaphane 8 units before bed.

He is not taking any other medicines.

His blood glucose appears to be well controlled, ranging between 6 and 9 mmol/L.

He has no health problems besides diabetes. He meditates daily to manage stress and keep life balance and is committed to maintaining his health and to self-care.

He is seeking advice about using Chinese medicine as part of his diabetes management plan.

Diabetes educator

Stress management techniques such as meditation have positive psychological benefits (see Chapter 8) and secondary benefits for blood glucose control by managing counter-regulatory hormone responses that contribute to hyperglycaemia. Stress management helps maintain a positive attitude, which is associated with improved immunity, coping, and resilience, which are all important aspects of managing diabetes. Mr AD is only 20 and these positive strategies will help him cope with diabetes in the long term and may prevent diabetes burnout.

I would ask him why he is interested in using Chinese medicine and which particular aspect of Chinese medicine he is thinking about using. He has type 1 diabetes, so glucose-lowering medicines are not indicated. However, these are only one modality commonly used in Chinese medicine. Other modalities such as diet, exercise, and meditation may be beneficial. Non-pharmacological pain management strategies such as acupuncture are useful, if pain was a concern.

CASE DISCUSSION

Ms HCM

Ms HCM was referred to an endocrinologist for investigation and management of hypoglycaemia
Ms HCM is a 30-year-old Chinese woman living permanently in Australia for the past 6 years. She has no known previous illnesses and is not taking any prescribed medicines. She recently returned from a visit to her mother in China. She presented to her general practitioner reporting episodes of sweating and loss of consciousness. The episodes were of recent onset, relatively unpredictable and were very frightening because she lived alone.

The doctor could find no physical causes for the episodes but felt that symptoms were consistent with an insulinoma and ordered some blood tests including random glucose and insulin and referred her to an endocrinologist for assessment.

The blood tests showed a 'very high insulin level' and a normal blood glucose (3 mmol/L) fasting. The endocrinologist repeated the insulin, C-peptide, and glucose levels and conducted a mixed meal test. These investigations revealed very high insulin levels corresponding with a high C-peptide, which coincided with hypoglycaemia symptoms and low blood glucose levels (< 3 mmol/L). An episode was witnessed in hospital during the mixed meal test. A CT of the abdomen was normal. The C-peptide level indicated the insulin was endogenous and Ms HCM was not injecting insulin.

Ms HCM was asked 'Do you take any alternative medicines or supplements?' to which she replied 'no'.

However, considering Ms HCM's Chinese background the question was reworded to 'Have you recently started taking any Chinese herbs or medicines to improve your health?' She then responded that her mother was concerned about her lack of energy and suggested she needed more 'fire' to bring her back into balance. Her mother had type 2 diabetes, which she controlled using diet, Tai Chi and Chinese herbal medicine. The medicine was prescribed to correct her yin/yang imbalance associated with diabetes.

The mother gave some of her herbal medicines to Ms HCM, which she had been taking ever since. The symptoms resolved when the herbal medicine was stopped.

Diabetes educator

Ms HCM's story adequately demonstrates the need to ask people about CAM use. Her history should have indicated the possibility she may have been using CAM and more effective questioning and active listening would have saved her a great deal of anxiety, unnecessary and expensive tests, and arrived at the diagnosis much sooner. The hypoglycaemia must have been very difficult to cope with and it is fortunate she did not have an accident or suffer trauma during a hypoglycaemic event.

Her story is also a salutatory message to health professionals who believe CAM glucose-lowering medicines do not work, given her endogenous insulin production and the resultant hypoglycaemia.

CASE DISCUSSION

> **Miss CP**
>
> ***Miss CP self-referred to a diabetes educator for advice***
> I have had type 2 diabetes for 8 years and I take metformin and Diamicron (gliclazide) every day. I go to the gym four times a week and I am about 52 kg but I still have the midriff fat. I read in a magazine recently that a new product that contains white kidney beans, chromium picolinate and bitter orange can help with weight and blood glucose control.
>
> I would appreciate more information please.
>
> I am interested in natural health care. My doctor told me I have borderline diabetes.
>
> Can I continue to take glucosamine for my arthritis?
>
> Will it affect my blood glucose?

Complementary therapist

There are two key issues to consider: the safety of glucosamine and its efficacy. Glucosamine is a naturally occurring substance that is required for the production of various substances that make up joint tissue such as articular cartilage, tendons and synovial fluid (Braun and Cohen 2007). It has chondroprotective and anti-inflammatory activities, which appear to be the result of multiple mechanisms working together and there is strong evidence that it is effective in providing relief from some of the symptoms of osteo-arthritis as well as being effective in slowing the disease progression (Towheed *et al.* 2005).

Although many different forms of glucosamine are available, most clinical studies have tested glucosamine sulphate, which shows positive results. In particular, a specific patented oral formulation of glucosamine sulphate from Rottapharm, Italy, which is available as a prescription medicine in Europe, has produced the most consistent results. A 2006 Cochrane systematic review that analysed the results of 20 clinical studies identified that non-Rotta preparations failed to produce benefits in pain and function whereas the Rotta-brand glucosamine sulphate was effective (Towheed *et al.* 2005).

Besides offering patients with osteoarthritis (OA) significant symptomatic relief and long-term joint protection, glucosamine is widely considered to be safe. Currently, no serious or fatal side effects have been reported for glucosamine, in contrast to NSAIDs, which are also widely used for the symptomatic relief of OA (Anderson *et al.* 2005).

While some preliminary evidence suggests glucosamine may cause changes in glucose metabolism and insulin secretion similar to those seen in type 2 diabetes in both rats and humans, these findings have been disputed and to date clinical studies in humans have not demonstrated an effect on glucose metabolism (Tannis *et al.* 2004; Anderson *et al.* 2005).

My recommendation to Miss CP would be to continue taking glucosamine because it is safe and effective. It would seem prudent to monitor blood glucose levels if she stops using it or increase the dose to identify whether the product affects her blood glucose levels.

Diabetes educator

It is important to stress to Miss CP that diabetes is a serious disease and she does not have 'borderline diabetes.' She is obviously making an effort to actively manage her diabetes and is eating an appropriate diet and exercising, which will benefit both her diabetes and her OA.

I am not familiar with the combination product Miss CP referred to and would ask her to bring the information to a subsequent meeting so I could find out more information for her from a CAM colleague. Bitter orange is often used in weight loss formulas to stimulate the gastrointestinal system. It may increase temperature, induce heart irregularities and increase the blood pressure. It may increase blood levels of many conventional medicines because it inhibits the P450-3A system. Bitter orange formulas should be used with care at the lowest dose and not used continuously. A proposed mechanism of action is that the amines in bitter orange stimulate beta 3 cell receptors to break down fat (in high doses) and increase the metabolic rate and possibly reduce appetite (Preuss 2002). It may have a similar effect to ephedrine on the central nervous system.

CASE DISCUSSION

> **Mrs THZ**
>
> ***Mrs THZ self-referred to a diabetes educator for advice***
> I have been reading about herbs to treat diabetes on the internet.
>   Can you tell me which ones are safe to use?
>   Do they work?
>   Where should I get them?

Complementary therapist

I would discuss three key points with Mrs THZ:

- the reliability of internet information and how to make decisions about its value and veracity;
- herbal medicine efficacy in relation to diabetes; and
- herbal medicine safety.

The internet is both a blessing and curse when it comes to health care information. Some sites contain information written by health care professionals, which is very useful and accurate, whereas other sites contain information that is merely advertisements. My first suggestion is to find a registered herbalist or naturopath who specialises in herbal medicine and discuss this topic with them.

Herbal medicine, sometimes known as phytotherapy, can be broadly defined as the science and art of using botanical medicines to prevent and treat illness and the study and investigation of these medicines. Many herbal medicines have been investigated under randomised controlled trial conditions and found to have significant pharmacological blood glucose-lowering effects. Herbal medicines such as fenugreek (*Trigonella foenum*), ivy gourd (*Coccinia indica*), American ginseng (*Panax quinquefolius*), *Gymnema sylvestre* and bitter melon (*Momordica charantia*) have been shown to lower blood glucose levels in clinical trials (Yeh *et al.* 2005). In addition, some herbal medicines have been shown to improve peripheral circulation, such as ginkgo biloba and horse chestnut extract (Braun 2007).

As with all medicines, the expected therapeutic benefits must be weighed against the potential risks. Some herbal medicines can cause significant drug interactions and adverse reactions, but when used correctly under the guidance of a knowledgeable health care professional, the risks can be minimised. In the case of using hypoglycaemic herbal medicines, professional supervision and frequent self-monitoring are advised to ensure that the intended outcome is achieved in a safe way.

Diabetes educator

These points are all very important. I would also explain that most of the trials of herbal medicines are in type 2 diabetes. It is not clear whether Mrs THZ actually has diabetes, and if so, what type she has or whether she is on any conventional medicines or uses other CAM. I would also advise her to inform her conventional health professionals if she does decide to use CAM.

References

Anderson JW, Nicolosi RJ, Borzelleca JF (2005) Glucosamine effects in humans: a review of effects on glucose metabolism, side effects, safety considerations and efficacy. *Food Chemical Toxicology* 43(2): 187–201.

Bakker SJL, Bilo HJG (2006) Chromium treatment has no effect in patients with poorly controlled, insulin-treated type 2 diabetes in an obese western population: a randomized, double-blind, placebo-controlled trial. *Diabetes Care* 29: 521–525.

Bjelakovic G, Nikolova D, Gluud LL *et al.* (2007) Mortality in randomised trials of antioxidant supplements for primary and secondary prevention. Systematic review and meta-analysis. *Journal of the American Medical Association* 297: 842–857.

Braun L (2006) Complementary medicine and safety. Chapter 3 in Dunning T (ed) *Complementary Therapies in the Management of Diabetes and Vascular Disease: A Matter of Balance*. Wiley and Sons, Oxford, pp 36–47.

Braun L, Cohen M (2007) Herbs and Natural Supplements – An Evidence-based Guide (2nd edn). Elsevier, Sydney.

Di Vincenzo R (2006) Nutritional therapies. Chapter 5 in Dunning T (ed) *Complementary Therapies in the Management of Diabetes and Vascular Disease: A Matter of Balance*. Wiley and Sons, Oxford, pp 77–146.

Egede L, Xiaobou Y, Zheng D *et al.* (2002) The prevalence and pattern of complementary and alternative medicine use in individuals with diabetes. *Diabetes Care* 25: 324–329.

Egger G, Cameron-Smith D, Stanton R (1999) The effectiveness of popular non-prescription weight loss supplements. *Medical Journal of Australia* 171: 604–608.

Faraday X (2006) American Heart Association Session, Abstract 4104, Chicago, November 14.

Grant P (2004) Warfarin and cranberry juice: an interaction? *Heart Valve Disease* 13(1): 25–26.

Gunton JE, Cheung NW, Hitchman R *et al.* (2005) Chromium supplementation does not improve glucose tolerance, insulin sensitivity, or lipid profile: a randomised placebo-controlled double blind trial of supplements in subjects with impaired glucose tolerance. *Diabetes Care* 28(30): 712–713.

Kleefstra N, Houweling ST, Jansman FG *et al.* (2006) Chromium treatment has no effect in patients with poorly controlled, insulin treated type 2 diabetes in an obese western population: a randomised double-blind, placebo-controlled trial. *Diabetes Care* 29: 521–525.

Kumar D, Bajaj S, Mehrotra R (2006) Knowledge, attitudes and practice of complementary and alternative medicines for diabetes. *Public Health* 120: 705–711.

Liu S, Lee I-M, Song Y *et al.* (2006) Vitamin E and risk of type 2 diabetes in the women's health study randomised controlled trial. *Diabetes* 55: 2856–2862.

Lloyd P, Lupton D, Wiesner D *et al.* (1993) Choosing alternative therapy: an Australian study of sociodemographic characteristics and motives of patients resident in Sydney. *Australasian Journal of Public Health* 17(2): 135–144.

McCarty M (1995) Anabolic effects of insulin on bone suggests a role for chromium picolinate in preservation of bone density. *Medical Hypotheses* 45(3): 241–246.

McKay D (2007) Vitamin E supplementation. An update. *Alternative Medicine Alert* 10(4): 37–42.

Natural Medicines Comprehensive Database (2006) (www.natural-database.com).

Preuss HG, Wallerstedt D, Talpur N *et al.* (2000) Effects of niacin-bound chromium and grape seed proanthacyanidin extract on the lipid profile of hypercholesterolemic subjects: a pilot study. *Journal of Medicine* 31(5–6): 227–246.

Preuss HG, DiFerdinando D, Bagchi M *et al.* (2002) *Citrus aurantium* as a thermogenic, weight-reduction replacement for ephedra: an overview. *Journal of Medicine* 33(1–4): 247–264.

Saltzman JR, Kemp JA, Golner BB *et al.* (1994) Effect of hypochlorhydria due to omeprazole treatment or atopic gastritis on protein-bound vitamin B12 absorption. *Journal of American College of Nutrition* 13(6): 584–591.

Tannis AJ, Barban J, Conquer JA (2004) Effect of glucosamine supplementation on fasting and non-fasting plasma glucose and serum insulin concentrations in healthy individuals. *Osteoarthritis and Cartilage* 12(6): 506–511.

Towheed TE, Maxwell L, Anastassiades TP *et al.* (2005) Glucosamine therapy for treating osteoarthritis. *Cochrane Database of Systematic Reviews* 2. CD002946. DOI: 10.1002/14651858.CD002946.pub2.

Vincent C, Furnham A (1997) Complementary medicine. A research perspective. *Medicine, Health Care and Philosophy* 1(2): 190–191.

World Health Organization (WHO) (2002) *Traditional Medicine Strategy 2002–2005*. WHO, Geneva.

Yeh GY, Eisenberg DM, Kaptchuk TJ *et al.* (2003) Systematic review of herbs and dietary supplements for glycemic control in diabetes. *Diabetes Care* 26(4): 1277–1294.

Recommended reading

Braun L, Cohen M (2006) *Herbs and Natural Supplements*. Elsevier, Sydney.

Dunning T (2006) *Complementary Therapies in the Management of Diabetes and Vascular Disease: A Matter of Balance*. Wiley and Sons, Oxford.

Index

Page numbers in *italics* refer to figures and those in **bold** refer to tables.